Contents

Chapter 1: What is Addiction?

Chapter 2: Addictions

Chapter 3: Help & Recovery

Introduction

Addiction is Volume 410 in the **issues** series. The aim of the series is to offer current, diverse information about important issues in our world, from a UK perspective.

ABOUT Addiction

Addiction can take many forms. As many as 1 in 3 people have an addiction to something. This book explores some of the common addictions affecting young people in the UK today, such as addictions to technology, caffeine and sugar. It also looks at why people become addicted and ways to overcome addiction.

OUR SOURCES

Titles in the **issues** series are designed to function as educational resource books, providing a balanced overview of a specific subject.

The information in our books is comprised of facts, articles and opinions from many different sources, including:

♦   Newspaper reports and opinion pieces

♦   Website factsheets

♦   Magazine and journal articles

♦   Statistics and surveys

♦   Government reports

♦   Literature from special interest groups.

A NOTE ON CRITICAL EVALUATION

Because the information reprinted here is from a number of different sources, readers should bear in mind the origin of the text and whether the source is likely to have a particular bias when presenting information (or when conducting their research). It is hoped that, as you read about the many aspects of the issues explored in this book, you will critically evaluate the information presented.

It is important that you decide whether you are being presented with facts or opinions. Does the writer give a biased or unbiased report? If an opinion is being expressed, do you agree with the writer? Is there potential bias to the 'facts' or statistics behind an article?

ASSIGNMENTS

In the back of this book, you will find a selection of assignments designed to help you engage with the articles you have been reading and to explore your own opinions. Some tasks will take longer than others and there is a mixture of design, writing and research-based activities that you can complete alone or in a group.

FURTHER RESEARCH

At the end of each article we have listed its source and a website that you can visit if you would like to conduct your own research. Please remember to critically evaluate any sources that you consult and consider whether the information you are viewing is accurate and unbiased.

Useful Websites

www.eandt.theiet.org

www.actiononaddiction.org.uk

www.bath.ac.uk

www.castlecraig.co.uk

www.drugwise.org.uk

www.healthandcare.scot

www.hebrontrust.org.uk

www.independent.co.uk

www.inews.co.uk

www.metro.co.uk

www.Pamela-Roberts.co.uk

www.prospectmagazine.co.uk

www.psychreg.org

www.rehab-online.org.uk

www.telegraph.co.uk

www.theconversation.com

www.thefoodaddictioncoach.co.uk

www.themix.org.uk

www.topdoctors.co.uk

www.ukactive.com

www.verywellmind.com

www.welldoing.org

www.yougov.co.uk

Addiction

What is addiction?

According to UK charity Action on Addiction, 1 in 3 people are addicted to something. Addiction is a complex brain disease where a person compulsively needs to use or take something that has a harmful consequence. Their intense focus on using a substance can take over their life even if they know that their constant use of a drug or alcohol, for example, can cause problems.

Changes in the brain's wiring are what make it difficult for a person to stop using or craving the substance that they are addicted to.

What can people be addicted to?

Besides addiction to toxic substances, such as alcohol and drugs, there are addictions of other types, such as:

♦ Food

♦ Cigarettes

♦ Sex (nymphomania)

♦ Gambling

♦ Exercise (bigorexia)

♦ New technologies (technophilia)

♦ Mobile phone use (nomophobia)

♦ Social media

For each individual case, professionals decide on the best treatment, depending on the patient's symptoms and the degree of their addiction.

What are the symptoms of addiction?

The symptoms of addiction can be broken down into three categories:

Psychological symptoms

♦ The inability to stop using

♦ Continual use of substances despite other health concerns

♦ Taking drugs or alcohol to deal with problems

♦ Obsessed with a substance

♦ Risk-taking or reckless behaviour - using sex to pay for drugs or stealing, or driving whilst under the influence

♦ Developing a tolerance and needing to take a higher dosage

Social symptoms

♦ Social isolation or distancing from friends who don't engage in drugs or alcohol

♦ Dropping hobbies

♦ Selling homely possessions in order to keep up drug supplies

♦ Denial

♦ Legal issues, such as being arrested

♦ Financial trouble

Physical symptoms

♦ Withdrawal symptoms

♦ Appetite changes, which leads to weight loss or gain

♦ Diseases, such as lung cancer from smoking hard drugs like crack or heavy nicotine use

♦ Insomnia

♦ A change in appearance.

What causes addictions?

Addiction can occur if someone is using drugs or alcohol to self-medicate any psychological pain felt from any traumatic experiences, such as a divorce, the death of a loved one or facing bankruptcy.

Because drugs and alcohol can affect the way that you feel and make you feel enjoyable and relaxed but after you 'come down' from these effects you can be left needing to recreate those feelings again, which creates a vicious cycle of taking more.

In cases of gambling, having a huge win can leave you feeling 'high' and that you want to win more, which can soon develop into a bad habit. An addiction gets out of hand when someone wants to continuously chase that high and feeling of euphoria.

How can someone get help for an addiction?

Addiction is a treatable condition and can be reversed. You can visit your GP for recommendations. There are many services across the UK that help people to recover from addiction. You can also speak to the Samaritans for free on 116 123 for advice.

If you are admitted to a treatment program, you might stay as an inpatient in a rehabilitation centre. If you are an outpatient you may attend daily group and individual therapy sessions.

Cognitive behavioural therapy (talking therapy) is used to help overcome addiction.

Specialists can help you to detox from drugs and provide medicines to help, such as methadone for someone who is coming off of heroin.

www.topdoctors.co.uk

What is addiction?

You can become addicted to literally anything - from Olivia Rodrigo to alcohol, there really is no discrimination when it comes to addiction. Uncovering the reasons why can be slightly more tricky though. Let's figure it out together by understanding what exactly addiction is.

Let's admit it. Life can become a bit repetitive sometimes. When you're not bored, you're probably stressed and so the cycle continues. Thank you, responsibility. So it's not really a shock that young people get the occasional urge to bypass reality and indulge in 'fun stuff' like sex, shopping, drinking, taking drugs, gambling, or even computer games.

But when does indulgence become dependence? And are some people more likely to become addicts than others?

Addiction meaning

Addiction is a compulsion to use a substance, or persist with certain behaviour to ensure you feel good – or to avoid feeling crappy. An addiction falls into two categories: physical and psychological. It doesn't even have to be a serious problem to be classed as an addiction. It can be any severity of addiction meaning anywhere from 'mild addiction' to 'serious addiction'.

♦ **Physical addiction** occurs after you take a substance so much it actually alters your body's chemistry. This means your body develops a hunger for this drug that you have to keep feeding. If you don't, your body goes into withdrawal and you get all kinds of nasty symptoms until you feed it again.

♦ **Psychological addiction** is when your brain gets hooked to a particular substance or behaviour that 'rewards' it, i.e., makes you feel good. Kinda crazy right? An addicted brain can actually produce physical manifestations of withdrawal, including cravings, irritability, insomnia, and depression. The mind is truly a powerful thing.

When it comes to alcohol, nicotine and illegal drugs, it's possible to develop either a physical addiction, psychological addiction, or a mixture of both.

Why/how do you become an addict?

Anyone who takes enough of a certain substance is at risk of becoming addicted to it. But people don't usually overindulge in a particular substance when they're living their best life. Most of the time there are underlying difficulties in an addict's life that caused the addiction. This could be trauma in the family, abuse, neglect, trouble at school/work, or even self-esteem issues.

You might be wondering, what is addiction? Good news, it's actually quite a logical process (all the STEM students, we're looking at you to help us out). If something gives you positive reinforcement, of course you're going to want to do it/take it again. It gives you pleasure, it's fun, it's enjoyable. The problem starts when you repeat the behaviour to get rid of a shitty feeling, and your life begins to revolve around it.

Are some people more susceptible to addiction to others?

The phrase 'addictive personality' gets thrown around a lot but it has no scientific basis. 'I like to tell clients that addiction is a great leveller,' says Dr Robert Hill, a consultant clinical psychologist. 'No one is immune. Anyone can become an addict.'

BUT there are a few factors that can lead to addiction. There's a genetic susceptibility to alcohol, and therefore alcoholism is likely to run in a family. This doesn't mean you're automatically going to be an alcoholic if a family member is one, but the risk is higher.

Being young is another contributor. Teenagers and people in their early 20s usually experiment with high-risk activities like drinking and drugs. Young brains aren't wired to think about the long-term consequences of their substance abuse, which can make them more likely to overindulge.

Although there isn't such a thing as an 'addictive personality', people who are sensation-seekers are generally more likely to experiment and can develop addictive behaviours. Poverty can also be a factor, as is growing up in an environment where other people are addicts.

'The main component is an intolerance of experiencing your emotions and being in the present,' says Dr Hill. 'There's an impatience to change one's mental or physical state. But no personality "type" is protected from addiction.'

What is addiction and what are the signs?

Although all different types of personalities and people can develop all types of addictions, the warning signs usually follow the same pattern, and include:

♦ An unhealthy focus on pursuing the substance/behaviour

♦ Excluding other activities that aren't related to using

♦ Going out primarily to use

♦ Needing more of the substance/behaviour to get the same high

♦ Disregard for other areas of your life including relationships, your health, or career

♦ Withdrawal symptoms if substance/behaviour is prohibited

If it's you who has an addiction, or a family member or friend, there's help out there. You can always reach out to our free support services as well as the resources we have on our website. There are so many addiction treatment options, including behavioural therapies and more. You just have to take the first step and reach out.

Recognising you have an addiction is a seriously difficult thing to do. It's an enormous step but once you've done it, you're on your way to recovery.

5 August 2021

Is there really such thing as having an addictive personality?

What compels one person to want to use drugs again and another not to bother has a lot to do with previous life experience.

By Ian Hamilton

We've all heard the term 'addictive personality' used to describe that compulsion for chocolate, alcohol or even binge-watching a TV series.

Officially, psychiatry doesn't recognise the term as a formal diagnosis. But there is clearly a difference between the way people manage their relationship with drugs, gambling and other potentially addictive behaviours. Some can take it or leave it, while others have less control over how much time and energy they spend on an activity or substance.

It's this difference that's fascinating to unpick. It reveals why some people are seemingly unable to control their drug use while others can. Even drugs like heroin or crack cocaine that we think of as highly addictive don't render every user as a slave to repeated use. Conscripted American soldiers in Vietnam used heroin for months during the war but most were able to stop using the drug when they returned home. Although this is an unusual situation, it does suggest that addiction is about much more than just the chemical.

So, what is it that compels one person who tries a drug like heroin to want to use it again and another not to bother? It would be tempting, although somewhat damning, to think it was simply down to genetics. Research supports this idea but at best only accounts for 50 per cent of the potential risk of addiction. In other words, if your parents had an addiction there is a one in two chance you will.

Like many aspects of genetics, this has an obvious flaw. We are more than just a skeleton filled with genes. The way our parents or those around us behave influences what we do. If we learn that the way to control anger, low mood or anxiety is by having a drink then there's a good chance we'll replicate that behaviour.

This interaction between nature and nurture is where the science is at right now. The good news is that addiction isn't entirely predetermined by genes. The bad news is that a combination of inheritance and how you grow up does increase the risk of developing unhealthy habits, whether that's with drugs, sex or food. Experiencing trauma such as emotional, psychological or sexual abuse is the common thread of people who develop drug dependence, but it by no means explains everyone's route into addiction.

Critically, it's that first experience with a substance that can produce a feeling people have rarely if ever have felt. Warmth, contentment or even excitement are all common features reported by those who go on to use again and again. This is when free will or choice is so severely compromised that it, in effect, vanishes. To the onlooker, this appears to be self-destructive but paradoxically the person repeating this pattern is trying to maintain psychological survival.

Gender also plays a role. Men are typically attracted to risk, whereas women are often trying to treat a pre-existing psychological issue. That's why men are over seven times more likely than women to be addicted to gambling. For drugs, the amount of time between the first use of a drug to the development of a problem is much shorter for women than men. An example of a clear gender difference but also one that we still don't have enough evidence to explain.

This isn't about personality traits such as being an introvert or extrovert; these characteristics are present whether you have an addiction or not. What seems to load the dice is previous life experience. Even then, that doesn't explain everyone's destiny.

There's still so much we don't know about why some people exhibit these compulsive behaviours and what maintains them. What we do know is that there is no 'type' of person that develops an addiction, they are as varied as the human characteristics that distinguish us from one another, reassuring and humbling in equal measure.

Ian Hamilton lectures in mental health at the Department of Health Sciences, University of York

8 August 2020

Is addiction a disease or a choice? We ask healthcare workers

A plurality of healthcare workers see willpower as the most important component in addiction, but most believe there are also factors outside individual control.

By Matthew Smith, Head of Data Journalism

How far can people control their addictions? Treating drug and alcohol misuse costs the NHS as much as £4 billion a year, so finding the answer could have a huge financial benefit.

As things stand, a previous YouGov study of the general population found that 44% of Britons believe people have a large amount of control over their addictions. Only 21% think people have little to no control over their behaviour.

But what do healthcare professionals think? A new YouGov study conducted among 1,027 health workers, including doctors, nurses and NHS staff, reveals to what extent they feel drug, alcohol and cigarette addiction and obesity are within the power of individuals to control.

Almost a third (31%) believe that cigarette addiction is entirely down to personal choice, with 16-20% saying the same of obesity and drug and alcohol addiction. By contrast, a mere 1-2% said these issues are completely outside of an individual's control.

Broadening the categories finds that 40-61% say that personal choice is a greater factor in these issues than things an individual can't help, like genetics. Only 12-19% take the opposite view, saying that such factors have a greater influence than personal choice.

Between 27% and 37% felt that both factors played an equally large role in addiction and obesity.

Most professionals accept that factors a person can't control play a role in addiction

However, looking at the data from a different perspective shows that the overwhelming majority of healthcare professionals (66-82%) believe that factors beyond a person's control play at least some role in addiction. In the case of obesity and drug and alcohol addiction 49-57% of professionals believe that the factors that are beyond the ability of a person to control are as big, if not bigger, than the willpower factor.

The NHS itself seems to be non-committal on how far it thinks addiction is within the ability of an individual's control, saying simply that 'Some studies suggest addiction is genetic, but environmental factors, such as being around other people with addictions, are also thought to increase the risk.'

31 January 2020

Do healthcare professionals see addiction as a matter of willpower, or is it beyong an individual's control?

When it comes down to issues like addiction and obesity, do you believe the reasons why people find themselves in these situations tends to be down to personal choice (e.g. the behaviour could be different if the person was willing to change) or due to factors beyond an individual's control (e.g. the behaviour is dictated more by genetics, upbringing etc)?
% of 1,027 healthcare professionals

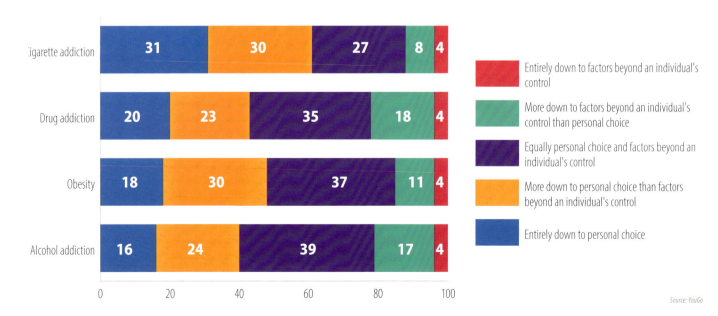

Source: YouGo

Why we become addicted

Addiction has to start somewhere. It begins with exposure, moves on to casual use and eventually turns to dependence. The brain adapts to the drug activity, becomes tolerant to it and demands more each time.

But not everyone becomes addicted. It's estimated that two million people in the UK are currently fighting an addiction. Many people drink or use drugs casually, but only some become psychologically dependent.

Great progress had been made in recent years in understanding why that is. Scientific research is beginning to understand the mechanisms in the addictive process, but we do not know exactly what causes addiction, or how to identify people who are likely to develop addictions.

'It seems to touch the very essence of behaviour, making it very difficult to research and understand,' said Ilana Crome, a professor of addiction psychiatry at Keele University.

Science cannot point to a 'single cause' of why addictions develop. Yet despite the difficulty in pinpointing exactly what makes some people more prone to addiction than others, countless studies have found that a combination of factors can play a part. Our environments, family backgrounds, personality traits, and even our genetics can all make someone more likely to try drugs or alcohol in the first place.

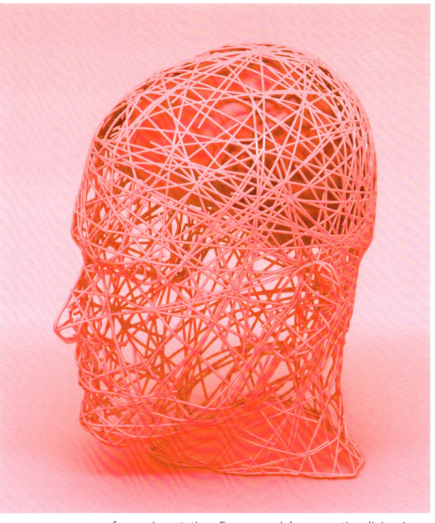

Some research suggests people who are prone to addiction may be 'wired' differently, particularly in the brain's orbito-frontal cortex.

'This part of the brain is involved in the weighing up of the pros and cons of a particular action, in other words, decision making,' explained Dr Owen Bowden-Jones, the chair of the Faculty of Addictions at the Royal College of Psychiatrists.

Psychological trauma is a common factor, he added. This could be anything from traumatic childhood experiences to experiencing bereavement.

A study carried out in 2012 also found that those with 'negative emotionality' have higher rates of drug abuse. This is a personality trait that dictates how intensely people experience dark emotions such as anger, stress or sadness.

According to the National Institutes of Health (NIH), the risk of addiction also increases for those who have parents who are/were alcoholics or drug addicts. It has been stated that the children of addicts are 45% to 79% more likely to abuse drugs or alcohol compared to the general population. It's unknown whether this is because addiction is rooted in genetics, if it's inherited, or if being exposed to drug taking and alcohol abuse increases the likelihood of experimentation. From a social perspective, living in an environment where drugs are easily available and their use normalised, or being surrounded by people who have addiction issues, is often cited as a common factor in the early exposure to – and subsequent dependence on – the substance or activity.

Those who live with mental health conditions such as bipolar disorder or depression are more likely to engage in substance abuse, which puts them at a higher risk of developing an addiction.

However, there are clearly many cases which do not fit these risk factors. Some people grow up in alcoholic households yet never become addicted themselves. Some are not exposed to the substance or activity in early life at all but go on to develop an addiction.

That's why it is impossible for science to identify those most likely to become addicted, as it's such an individual thing. Many people who have experienced a difficult background or trauma who might be predicted to develop an addiction don't.

30 March 2022

Can you be addicted to dopamine?

By Ariane Resnick, CNC. Medically reviewed by Steven Gans, MD

Pleasure is something we all need in life. At times, though, we can get too focused on it, or on specific activities that feel pleasurable to us. They can get out of control, and may even lead to addiction. This is because we can get hooked on the good feelings we're flooded with when we conduct pleasurable activities.

Those feelings are often referred to as a 'high,' which is something people are known to 'chase.'

We'll take a look at the brain chemical dopamine and examine how it can be a slippery slope for some people in relation to addiction. First, you'll learn what dopamine is. Then, we'll examine the pleasurable activities that can provide it, why they can potentially lead to problems, and what behaviours you can follow to prevent getting too dependent on the feelings that accompany a surge in dopamine.

What is dopamine?

Dopamine is a neurotransmitter. That means it's a chemical that sends signals inside our brains. Neurotransmitters have a wide assortment of functions, and dopamine's function centres around the pleasure and reward areas of our brains.

It's known as one of the 'pleasure chemicals' because of that fact. Other feel-good chemicals include serotonin, oxytocin, and endorphins.

When you do something that you like the feeling of, your brain sends a signal of pleasure to your brain. Then, you associate that activity with the feeling of pleasure. When that happens, it can become difficult to separate the physical occurrence from the feeling of pleasure it gave you.

It's normal to then remember that experience as something that provided you with good feelings.

Dopamine is important in our everyday lives outside of feelings of pleasure. It plays a role in everything from motivation to mood to memory. Having a healthy level of dopamine is necessary, and if your body isn't producing enough, it can lead to problems such as depression and insomnia.

Activities that release dopamine

Basically, anything you do that feels good can release dopamine in your brain. Some of these things are good ways to naturally ensure you have sufficient dopamine levels, and some aren't. These are some examples of activities that release dopamine:

♦ Having sex

♦ Eating a tasty meal or dessert

♦ Exercise

♦ Listening to music

♦ Caffeine

♦ Recreational drugs and alcohol

♦ Meditation

Risky behaviours associated with dopamine

You may have heard the saying that it's possible to get too much of a good thing. That idea is why dopamine can potentially become a problem for someone.

Let's look at what becoming dependent on the rush of dopamine can involve.

Sex addiction

For one example, getting dependent on having sex can lead to sex addiction. Because it makes us feel good, we may seek it out in ways that are unsafe for us. This can involve having unprotected sex, having sex with someone who is a stranger and might be dangerous, or not taking care of the responsibilities you have in life because you are busy pursuing sex.

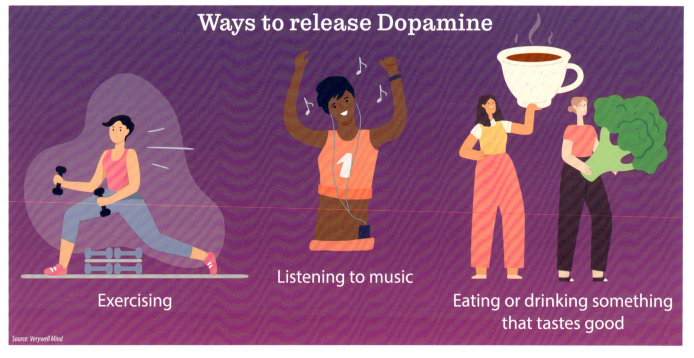

Ways to release Dopamine

Exercising

Listening to music

Eating or drinking something that tastes good

Source: Verywell Mind

Food-related disorders

Another example of risky behaviour that can be based in the urge for dopamine is eating. On the one hand, we have to eat! We can't survive without it. And it's completely normal to want to eat foods that taste good to us.

However, eating can get out of control and become a food addiction, in which a person's relationship with food becomes more about eating to feel good than eating to stay alive.

Alcohol and substance use disorders

A third example of how the quest for dopamine can lead to problems is with alcohol and recreational drugs. These substances release dopamine in the most straightforward way of all, with drugs like cocaine directly flooding our brains with it.

Drug addiction and alcoholism can be life-threatening and can have terrible impacts on the lives of both the person with the addiction and everyone else they are close to.

In addition to the above, there are countless other dopamine-oriented activities that can lead to major problems and risky behaviours. They can be as big and life-altering as losing your financial savings due to gambling, or as temporary as exercising too much and obtaining a minor injury from overusing parts of your body.

Is dopamine addiction possible?

It is not technically possible to get addicted to dopamine. It occurs naturally in our bodies, and we can't directly take it as a food or drug. However, it is completely possible to get addicted to any activity that increases our dopamine levels.

Even though we aren't directly addicted to dopamine itself, we may be addicted to an activity because of the dopamine it releases in our brains.

Ways to avoid dopamine dependence

Although it's important to perform activities that release dopamine, for the sake of feeling good regularly, it is also vital that you don't become dependent on that release.

It might be a shorter journey than you'd think to go from simply enjoying a pleasurable act on occasion and being hooked on it in a way that is harmful to your life (or the lives of others).

Below are some ideas to help you have a healthy relationship with dopamine and help avoid dependence.

Activity boundaries

In order to avoid getting too much of a good thing, it can be helpful to have boundaries. For example, if you love to

exercise but you find yourself getting hurt because you're overdoing it, set up your workout plan a week ahead of time.

Review your plan and consider confirming with a professional trainer that it is a moderate exercise plan and not one that risks you getting injured because it's too strenuous.

As far as how to set your boundaries, if you have a good memory you can simply think ahead and schedule out how long you'll spend with different activities or how much of them you'll do.

If you want to feel more accountable to yourself than that, or your memory isn't great, use a journal to write down your boundaries or send an email to yourself.

Nerve-calming practices

Making sure you are getting enough relaxation in your day can help to combat the feeling that you need to perform dopamine-boosting activities more often than what is considered healthy.

Any self care practice can be calming to your nerves, as can very simple activities like deep breathing.

Conduct activities mindfully

Another great way to keep tabs on yourself and avoid getting too dependent on the release of dopamine is to make yourself more aware of what you do.

Mindfulness is the act of making a big point of paying attention in the moment, day to day, rather than functioning on autopilot all the time.

Before you set out to do something you enjoy that you feel you might be getting dependent on, check in with yourself.

Assess how you're feeling, what you're thinking, and any concerns you may have about your behaviour. Then as you go along with that activity, continue checking in with yourself to make sure everything is feeling calm and not like you're getting too into the 'high' of the act.

What to do if things get out of control

Addiction is complex, and science is still uncovering why it affects some people more than others. Even though you can't be directly addicted to dopamine, you can get addicted to any activity that releases it.

If you've tried to mitigate your behaviour and you haven't been successful, there are many people who can help you.

29 November 2021

Seven things you're getting wrong about addiction

By Ellen Scott

Try as we might to be understanding and open-minded, many of us have some rigidly held beliefs when it comes to addiction.

And often, those beliefs are completely incorrect, built on outdated stereotypes and assumptions.

This is why addiction remains one of the most misunderstood mental health issues, despite hundreds of thousands of people in the UK suffering.

So, let's get debunking, so we can get a clearer picture of what addiction is actually like.

Ahead, the experts at Delamere and psychiatrist Dr Catherine Carney break down seven of the most common misconceptions about addiction, and explain the reality.

Myth: If you have a career and family, you can't suffer from addiction

There's a picture many of us have in our heads of what an addict looks like.

Often, this is a dishevelled man who's homeless or out of work.

Dr Catherine Carney says: 'The idea that those suffering from addiction are individuals who are homeless or out of work is a problematic stereotype that is false.

'In fact, many people suffering have families and a stable career.

'This is often labelled as a functioning addiction, which refers to someone who suffers from substance disorder but can still manage their daily lives and are very good at masking their issues.'

Myth: Addiction is just about drugs and alcohol

Yes, a lot of addiction is related to the abuse of drugs and alcohol, but there are other areas of addiction that we don't often think about.

What about gambling, overeating, sex, shopping?

Myth: Addiction is a bad choice people make

'To begin with, engaging in the misuse of a particular substance may seem to be a voluntary choice, but the way the brain reacts to the chemical is not,' explains Dr Catherine.

'Once a substance is misused regularly, it changes the brain's reaction to it each time it is used, which makes discontinuing a substance that a person is addicted to, challenging without professional help and support.'

Myth: Once an addict, always an addict

Recovery is possible.

Dr Catherine says: 'Though some people may suffer from addiction for a long period of time, many people do recover from their problems with the correct support and treatment.

'While initially seeking help may be a challenge, the right treatment facility and recovery programme can help those facing addiction overcome the challenges of addiction.

'However, the nature of addiction means that some people may relapse or return to drug use after attempting to stop or finishing treatment, but the most effective methods of help are often designed to support those who have relapsed.'

Myth: You don't need treatment until you hit rock bottom

'Waiting until you hit 'rock bottom' is actually a really dangerous myth surrounding addiction that could mean it's a more challenging process for recovery,' explains Dr Catherine.

'Everyone's version of rock bottom can be different so it is important to seek help as soon as you start to recognise the signs and symptoms of addiction.

'It's important to help family, friends and colleagues who are showing signs to seek professional help.

'Just because your symptoms may not be as severe as others yet, not seeking help when you need it can lead to more challenging consequences.'

Myth: Taking prescription pills is less addictive or dangerous than illegal drugs

If a doctor gave you medication, it must be safer than something you're getting off the street, right?

Not so much – you're just as able to become addicted. And in fact, Dr Catherine notes, addiction to prescription pills can be more complicated as it's harder to identify.

It can also be a gateway to other substances.

t

'Anyone can suffer from addiction and no one is exempt,' says Dr Catherine. 'It can affect all demographics and professions, so the more that people are aware of the signs and symptoms of addiction, the easier it will be to break down the stigma surrounding addiction.'

6 February 2022

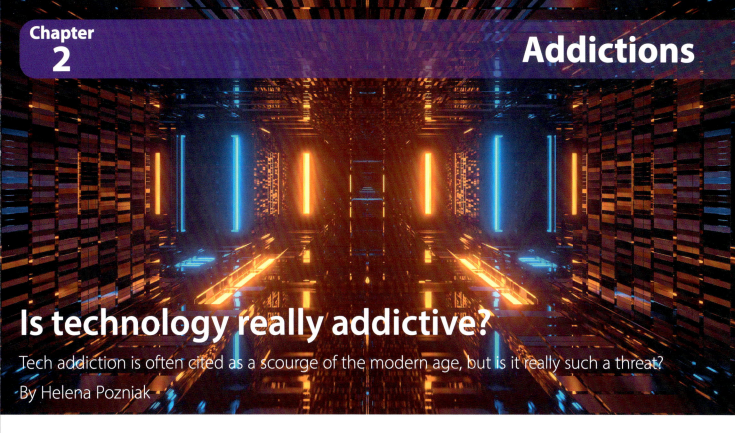

Is technology really addictive?

Tech addiction is often cited as a scourge of the modern age, but is it really such a threat?

By Helena Pozniak

D oes technology addiction really exist? And is it damaging us? Ask any parent whose adolescent child is chained to their device or obsessed by gaming into the small hours – and they'll agree. So too does the World Health Organization (WHO), which controversially classified 'gaming disorder' as a disease in 2018.

By talking about addiction, we're succumbing to 'techno-panic', say some psychologists – and many have publicly protested against WHO's decision.

Every age worries what its teens are up to – even comics and romance novels once sparked panic, says psychologist Candice Odgers, who's researched technology use among young people. Our current objections may be based upon weak data.

She's used to being accosted by angry parents since she pointed out research doesn't definitively link use of mobile devices and social media to mental health problems in young people.

A 2017 US study stirred widespread panic as reports declared adolescents spending more time on social media were more likely to report mental health issues. In fact, 'digital media use accounted for less than 1 per cent of the differences in depressive symptoms among girls, and no association was found among boys,' says Odgers. 'To be precise, 99.64 per cent of the differences in girls' depression was due to something else. Technology is as likely as, say, eating potatoes to cause mental health problems.'

> '**Behavioural addictions are harder to treat; normally we'd advise abstinence, but technology is inescapable today – you need it for work, everyone has a screen**'
>
> **Rebecca Sparkes, psychotherapist**

One of the largest studies so far, which looked at more than 120,000 adolescents in the UK, reported no association between moderate levels of technology use and mental health. In fact, devices could even lead to better wellbeing – although the research also noted small negative associations for people with high levels of engagement. What is going on?

Rates of depression and suicide are undoubtedly rising – not only among young people – and this requires urgent attention, psychologists agree. This year, the family of a 14-year-old girl who killed herself said images she had seen on Instagram were partly to blame, which has led the UK to consider a mandatory code of conduct for big tech companies.

How we spend our time undoubtedly differs from the pre-internet era – just look across a crowded train to witness a sea of devices where once there might have been readers, knitters and even chatters. UK teenagers are on their phones for about 18 hours a week – many for far longer – and much of that time is spent on social media. One in three internet users is a child. Parents fear online gaming, which some believe leads on to gambling – a recognised addiction, not to mention excessive use of social media, porn and harmful content. Are developing brains really safe from technology?

Recent media reports have claimed technology is as addictive 'as cocaine', but this is fear-mongering, writes Christopher Ferguson, professor of psychology at Stetson

University. Using technology activates roughly the same pleasure circuits as class A drugs – but so do many other pleasurable activities: from exercise, to eating, to sex. 'Technology use causes dopamine release similar to other normal fun activities: about 50 to 100 per cent above normal levels,' he writes. Cocaine on the other hand increases dopamine by 350 per cent; methamphetamine by 1,200 per cent.

Also, can tech users really be labelled as addicts? The NHS defines an addiction as not having control over doing, taking or using something to the point where it could be harmful. According to Action on Addiction, one in three are addicted to something. But withdrawing from technology use doesn't prompt the same acute physical symptoms as does quitting drugs or alcohol. Just 3 per cent of gamers develop problem behaviours, such as neglecting school work, and most of these problems eventually disappear, says Professor Ferguson.

A 2016 study found those who appear more addicted to games don't show more psychological or health problems. One of the most common research findings, says Odgers, is that children who struggle in their offline lives are those who have the most negative experiences online. 'Offline risk predicts online risk.'

But even if the problem is relatively mild, the ubiquity of technology makes it impossible to escape, says psychotherapist Rebecca Sparkes, who counsels addicts of all kinds. Losing sleep, not seeing friends, not being physically active is damaging. 'I have a coterie of young clients who're concerned how much of their time they're "losing" to online gaming. I'm incredibly concerned about it. Behavioural addictions are harder to treat; normally we'd advise abstinence, but technology is inescapable today – you need it for work, everyone has a screen.'

During treatment, says Dr Nick Maguire, associate professor of psychology at the University of Southampton, he'll ask addicts what level of insight they have about their addiction, and how motivated they are to tackle it – before looking at what function it serves in their lives and how the addiction might be treated. But social media and gaming often help those who might be struggling socially; it's hard to judge at what stage it might become problematic.

While there has been a flurry of research around our use of technology – including problem shopping, digital hoarding (hanging on to images, texts) and so on – science now needs to look with more detail at what young people are actually doing online, says Odgers.

Spending time learning online is obviously not the same as gaming or scrolling through Instagram, for instance, so researchers now need to ask better questions. Science is also hampered by a lack of a control group – but then, try finding a group of adolescents willing to give up their mobiles for any length of time.

A focus on addiction fears might mask potential benefits that technology offers, such as enhancing social relationships. If we become overly hung up on fears of addiction, will we see technology use wrongly – as a cause rather than a symptom of unhappiness – and perhaps miss the bigger picture? 'There's shockingly little good evidence on this topic,' says Odgers.

10 September 2019

Case Study: Gambling addiction

Gambling is recognised as an addiction, and ease of access through smartphone use has proved devastating. Those aged 25-34 account for the biggest increase in online gambling of any age group (Gambling Commission) and are most likely to hold more than five online gaming accounts. Former online gambler James says his addiction worsened after the death of his mother when he was 19. 'Amounts of money grew bigger and the time I spent on it every day just got worse and worse,' he says.

By the time he asked for help, he was 24, living in his car and suicidal. His father booked him into addiction clinic PCP, where he eventually quit. But last year, seven months clean, he relapsed. 'There was an ad on telly for (online gambling firm) Bet365,' he says. 'I signed up within three minutes and went on a spree that lasted two and a half days, until I ran out of money. With online gambling it's so easy, you don't value the money, it's easier to continue until you literally have nothing left.'

A close friend helped him back from the brink, and he's never gambled since. He now volunteers to help others. 'I've quit all my social media accounts because that's where I'd see ads for gambling, and I was constantly online – it's as if I was addicted to those too.' An early intervention programme may have saved him. 'If you can plant a seed at a young age that gambling is a problem, then you'd prevent many people going down that route in adulthood.'

Fears over technology 'addictions' and 'disorders' may be unjustified, shows research

Current measures of digital technology use are not fit for purpose, say University researchers.

Questionnaires and scales measuring how we interact with smartphones, social media and gaming should not be used to demonstrate links with mental health and wellbeing, according to research from the Universities of Bath and Lancaster.

Surveys that ask people about their technology habits often suggest problematic use, even pointing towards the potential for 'addictive' behaviours. But when researchers analysed these questionnaires, they found that these measures were not advanced enough to confirm any such issues.

Despite claiming to identify unique issues to specific technologies, such as phobias or addictions, many scales are related to each other. For example, if a participant scored highly on a smartphone 'addiction' survey they were also likely to score high on a scale that measured internet gaming 'disorder'.

'Many technology measures appear to identify a similar, poorly defined construct that sometimes overlaps with measures of well-being. However, we need more research to determine exactly what these scales measure,' said Dr Brit Davidson, from the University of Bath's School of Management.

Dr David Ellis, also from Bath's School of Management, added: 'Technology usage scales continue to be developed at an alarming rate and yet we now know their foundations are shaky. This only serves to distract from genuine online harms, including online harassment, misinformation, and data security.'

Published in *Computers in Human Behaviour* three separate studies analysed the function of the scales and set out to investigate precisely what they measure, analysing the Smartphone Addiction Scale, the Internet Gaming Disorder Scale, the Bergen Social Media Addiction Scale and the Problematic Series Watching Scale.

'The scales are not developed in line with best practices yet allow researchers to quickly link mental health symptoms to technology use,' said Dr Heather Shaw from the School of Psychology at Lancaster University.

Dr Davidson added: 'While our attention is focused on alarming headlines we are not putting energy into truly understanding the impact of digital technology. Findings involving these widely used scales continue to drive research agendas, inform policy and are even attempting to define new clinical disorders.'

The researchers say more research is needed to understand people's everyday experiences with digital technology alongside accurate measures of behaviour from gaming and social media platforms.

1 June 2022

Why are we so addicted to social media?

Social media holds an undeniable presence in most of our lives – but why is it that we find it so addictive? Teacher and trainee psychotherapist Emma Kilburn explores three different psychological theories to explain why we're hooked.

By Emma Kilburn

Over the last few months, many of us will have spent more time than ever in front of a screen. For those working from home, a lot of this time will have been dedicated to work-related activity. However, the period of lockdown also saw a sharp increase in the amount of screen time we spent socialising and keeping in touch with friends and family. It is hard to imagine how different our experience would have been had the pandemic struck pre-Facebook, WhatsApp, Instagram, Zoom or Houseparty. We would have experienced our physical isolation in a much more immediate way, without the technology and apps that enabled most of us to maintain contact with our support networks.

Our recent experiences have shone a fresh light on their undeniable benefits. Even in less extraordinary times, technology and in particular social networks can be very positive aspects of our daily lives. Of course, a great deal has also been written about the negative impact of the social media – in particular in terms of the amount of time we dedicate to them, and the psychological impact they can have. I have written previously about the pernicious impact of envy and how social media can fuel this and other negative emotions. Furthermore, research has shown that all kinds of comparisons via social media – whether we feel we are better or worse off than the people whose posts we are reading – can have a negative impact and can lead to depressive symptoms. Yet despite the possible psychological drawbacks – and despite our increasing awareness of the ways in which technology is being used to influence what we see in our feeds – social media networks continue to command as much of our time as ever. It is interesting to consider our relationship with these networks in the context of the work of theorists whose ideas may help us develop a clearer understanding of the drives that influence our decisions to dedicate so much time to them.

Why are we so addicted to social media?
#FOMO

The first reason social networks can be so addictive is linked to the acronym most closely associated with them: FOMO, or Fear Of Missing Out. Social networks create a sense of belonging and a sense of community. We build links with people who share the same interests and values as us by following them, re-tweeting them, or even by engaging with them directly. We are able to keep in contact with friends and colleagues with whom we might otherwise have lost touch, and can follow their lives online. We can participate and share in key events, whether that be the response to a sporting fixture, jokes and anger following the controversial actions of a public figure, or expressions of solidarity after

a natural disaster or a terrorist attack. We invest these connections with value and meaning. If we choose to step away from social media, these are lost and we are left wondering what connections and shared experiences people are having in our absence, while we remain on the outside of them. If we never engage with social media, these connections hold no value for us, but once we sign up, our FOMO makes it difficult for us to disengage, albeit we might manage to do so for a short period of time, encouraged by initiatives such as Scroll Free September.

Beyond shared experiences, social media networks draw us in due to the way in which they enable us to create and respond to social objects. A social object is an object that gains meaning through the way it is used. Internet entrepreneur Jyri Engestrom linked the success of key social networks to the way in which they extend the concept of sociality beyond people to social objects. People don't just connect to each other; they connect through a shared object, around which the conversations of social networks are generated. Photos on Flickr or Instagram, or videos on YouTube are all examples of social objects whose value lies in the way in which users engage with them, particularly since they are user-generated and so have no intrinsic value of their own. These objects constitute a key driver behind the time and emotional energy we choose to invest in social networks.

Validation

I have said that the value of social objects lies in the responses they generate, and this links to another key reason why social networks can be so addictive. Social media platforms encourage us to focus on the validation and recognition they can provide. If you post a picture on Instagram, your notifications will tell you how many people have liked it. The more the better, right?! If you tweet a response to an author, politician, or comedian on Twitter and they like your tweet, you feel proud, and seen. Perhaps you have sent a more negative comment to someone you disagree with, and have felt satisfied when they have engaged with what you have written, albeit perhaps in a similarly negative way.

The Swiss psychiatrist Eric Berne developed the concept of 'strokes.' He defined a stroke as the 'fundamental unit of social action'. Just as children want physical contact ('strokes'), adults need engagement, and these strokes can be symbolic, verbal or even digital, as well as physical. A physical stroke might be a hug, a verbal stroke a conversation, or even just a quick greeting. Strokes can be unconditional ('I think you are great') or conditional ('I think you are great, though not when we disagree on politics'.) They can be positive, or negative. Such is what Berne described as our 'recognition hunger' that even a negative stroke is better than no recognition at all, and this extends to our life online.

Our busy modern lives – or recently, the lockdown – often mean that we have fewer opportunities to engage with friends and family in person, and therefore fewer opportunities for physical or face-to-face contact and recognition. Social media offers us a virtual alternative through retweets, likes, shares, and even through negative interactions, since even this negative recognition goes some way towards sating our recognition hunger, despite the possible negative psychological consequences of disagreements, trolling and online hate-speak with which we may be left when we step away from our screens. Greater awareness of this psychological drive for recognition can help us understand why we are pulled to interact online, even when we may then be adversely affected by the consequences of our interactions. This might encourage us to seek a better balance between our face-to-face relationships and the time we spend on social media and to seek out more frequent opportunities for nurturing, real-life interactions with people we value. We may then feel less compelled to turn to social media in search of strokes, and thus avoid some of the psychological pitfalls of life online.

Comfort

A third theory that can help us understand the way in which we can become dependent on social media is linked to the device itself through which we most frequently access it, i.e. our mobile phone. This theory derives from the work of child psychologist D.W. Winnicott, who was active in the latter half of the twentieth century. Winnicott introduced the concept of the transitional object. This object allows a child to move from her initial, narcissistic view of the world in which it cannot see beyond itself, to an understanding of and love for others as complete people who are separate from the self. The transitional object is the first that become a focus of a child's attention and which enables her to develop an awareness of the self and other, while at the same time providing an ongoing source of security and comfort. Think about the soft toy you had as a child, or the blanket you had to cuddle or chew to soothe yourself to sleep - those were your transitional objects. Of course, over time, a child becomes more independent and equally becomes less emotionally invested in his or her transitional object. Nonetheless, that potential for emotional investment remains, and in later life other objects may fulfil the same role. In teenagers, we may see this emotional energy transferred to a pop star or actor for example, or to a particular cultural group or set of values. Objects in the cultural domain can be particularly effective transitional objects for young people as they offer scope for creativity, imagination and an exploration of potential self-fulfilment, since they are located in a potential space, somewhere between the inner world of the self and the external world of material reality.

Recently, various theorists have suggested that the mobile phone can play the role of transitional object. Much like a soft toy, mobile devices can provide a sense of comfort and familiarity in an unfamiliar setting. Sitting in a restaurant waiting for a friend, or attending a work conference with strangers, our mobile phone gives us a way to connect to social objects and to people that we know, so that we feel less alone or uncertain. Despite the known psychological risks associated with social media in particular, our phones can provide a means of escape from the place in which we are physically located, into a more familiar and comfortable psychic space, providing relief or release. Our phone enables us to move between the external world and our internal world. In this way it replicates the role of our Ego (in Freudian terms), whose main focus is to negotiate between the internal and external worlds, and to have its needs met in socially acceptable ways. Furthermore, the way we use our phone to connect with social media, to send emails or to search the internet enables us to create our own personalised experience, and in a way to reclaim the reassuring sense of narcissistic omnipotence we experienced as a very young child, before the presence of The Other made itself known.

In childhood, transitional objects enable us to manage the transition to a more structured existence, in which we have to manage our relationship with the other, and the passage of time. Similarly, our mobile phones can give our lives structure, via reminders and alarms, notifications, and a whole range of apps that remind us to keep 'doing' and 'planning' - whether those be fitness trackers, language learning apps, or simply notes containing our to-do list. The danger is when our phones become overly intrusive. Our to-do list turns our daily lives into a series of chores; our access to email enables our work life to intrude into our personal life; our constant need to be doing or updating distracts us and impedes our ability to just be, not least since regularly reaching for our phone fragments our focus and our experiences. And while our mobile phone and the access it gives us to social media can be a tool to enhance our relationships and provide a source of comfort to ward off any sense of alienation, the danger is that we may become overly dependent on our digital existence and miss the real thing.

I would by no means advocate that we should cease to engage with and use social media. It can bring many benefits, as long as we are aware of the potential pitfalls it presents, and if we take care to protect and nurture the life and relationships that we have built offline, in the real world. We should enjoy a gig, rather than watching it through our smartphone as we film it to share online. We should pause and appreciate a sunset, rather than seeking to capture and share it on Instagram. While we engage with our social networks we should aim to remember that the identity and life that we and others create on them can never be more than a partial representation of the more important and more complete lives and experiences that we are living on a daily basis.

21 September 2020

'Spiritual opium': could gaming addiction ruin a generation?

It's an industry worth billions but more than 86 million players have a dangerous obsession – and the pandemic has only made things worse.

By Annabel Heseltine

It will surely never happen again – but every parent must have been nodding in agreement with the Chinese state media yesterday. That's because it declared online games were 'spiritual opium… that has grown into an industry worth hundreds of billions… No industry, no sport, can be allowed to develop in a way that will destroy a generation.'

It's hard to disagree. In the past decade or so, online games have become ubiquitous around the world in a way that may be best described as careless.

From hailing the education potential of the internet, schools are now warning that classroom iPads and online textbooks are normalising the use of screens in a way which is potentially harmful to teenage brains. MRI scans have found the part of the brain which controls compulsive behaviour and decision-making tend to be less developed in teenagers who game for more than 10 hours a day.

Video games first emerged in the Fifties and Sixties, quickly shrinking in size to handheld consoles; the Nineties saw the Nintendo Gameboy challenging the Sega Game Gear for market dominance. Families began to share their TVs and homes with the Sega Mega Drive and Sony PlayStation – still sold as a fun, joint experience.

Yet, by the turn of the 21st century, as equipment became more sophisticated, graphics and storyboard quality improved with Hollywood actors lending their names and voices, another shift took place as young people got their own laptops or mobile phones and internet access exploded in range. Broadband – allowing telephone and computers to work at the same time – emerged. Initially download speeds were slow but in 10 years they escalated by a factor of 40 from 1.4mbps in 2012, according to Curry's, to 54.2mbps. Suddenly, games could be played – no more buffering – anywhere and anytime. So they were. And we parents enabled it.

A survey by the charity ChildWise revealed schoolchildren now spend an average of six hours a day in front of screens, while a separate report suggested the figure for teenagers is closer to 10 hours, with 43 per cent having internet access in their bedrooms.

It's a situation that worries novelist Abi Silver. When Covid hit and schools closed in March 2020, she had more reason than most for concern: her son Aron, now 17, had only just beaten a severe gaming addiction which had turned her family upside down for two years; now the computer would be his lifeline. 'His only contact with his friends was online and I wasn't going to deprive him of that,' says Silver, who is also a lawyer with her own consulting business.

The mother of two other sons, aged 19 and 21, Silver still wonders whether she could have done more to prevent him gaming. Together with her husband, Daniel, also a lawyer, she fought to keep technology out of the home. 'I didn't want them even to have mobile phones too early,' Silver says. 'But then it got to the stage in 2017 when they were saying: "If we don't have a PlayStation, Mum, nobody is going to come to our house".'

Aron, the youngest, was 13 at the time – bright, inquisitive, football-mad and a guitar player, but also shy. Silver, worrying about his social life, bowed to pressure. 'I didn't want him to feel excluded, so suddenly we had a PlayStation.'

The next thing she knew was their son had vanished into a room at the top of the house with his headphones on, was refusing to join family meals and shouting and arguing with his parents. 'There was a lot of resentment and accusations,' says Silver, 'I felt desperate.'

Five issues that hurt gamers

Sight

Spending less time outdoors and more time doing 'near work', like looking at screens and reading, is a cause of short-sightedness. A recent study shows that more screen time during the pandemic has led to a threefold increase in myopia in children in China.

Gamer's thumb aka Nintendonitis

Repetitive hand movements of tapping a smartphone screen or pressing buttons on a gaming console can cause inflammation of the tendons supporting the thumb. This painful condition is known as De Quervain syndrome and can limit movement in the hand.

Sleep

Research from 2014 found that gaming for more than an hour a day increased the risk of bad sleep quality by 30 percent. The bright light of a screen and excitement makes gaming in the evening a particular risk.

Obesity

Gaming can both increase the amount of time spent sitting down versus exercising, and increase mindless eating. A 2011 study found that participants ate significantly more while gaming than while resting, even though they did not report being hungry.

Posture

Spending long periods of time in one position, whether that's slouched in front of a monitor or hunched over a phone, can lead to pain and poor back strength.

Helen Chandler-Wilde

She adds: 'We tried to put limits on how much he could play but we ended up arguing with him. He needed a computer for homework so it was hard to know what he was doing.'

Then, in 2018, Aron discovered Fortnite, which a year on from production had amassed 80 million players, netting an annual profit of £5.5 billion for its manufacturer, Epic. Aron seemed obsessed with the addictive, dopamine-releasing game.

He was not alone. Parents everywhere were getting emails from their heads of schools warning of concerns over the game being highly addictive, opening up the potential to talk to strangers and encouraging children to run up large bills on their parents' bank accounts.

'Aron's head wanted us parents to talk to our children about it,' says Silver. 'I was shocked, and indignant, that there was something out there, unregulated and freely available to our kids, which was considered highly dangerous but nobody was doing anything about it. It was like someone was coming into my son's bedroom at night and injecting him with an addictive drug.'

Silver delved deeper, luckily able to turn for help to her elder sister, Naomi Fineman, professor of psychiatry at the University of Hertfordshire. For the past three years, Prof Fineman has chaired a global action group comprising scientists, doctors, psychologists and teachers researching Problematic Use of the Internet (PUI), including gambling, pornography, cyberbullying, social media and gaming.

Gaming addiction then became the subject of Silver's fifth book, *The Midas Game*, which sees two lawyers team up to defend a local gamer and YouTube celebrity who has been accused of killing an eminent anti-gaming psychiatrist. The subtext examines the responsibility of game manufacturers and the glamorising of gaming role models competing in high stakes e-sport leagues; last year, a 16-year-old gamer called Bugha won $3 million at the Fortnite World Cup.

Silver is appalled the industry is still unregulated, even though in 2018, the World Health Organisation classified 'gaming disorder' as an illness with, by their conservative estimate, some 86 million victims.

Post-lockdown, numbers are growing. 'The problem is that although a significant bank of research links high levels of online gaming with depression, social anxiety, suicidal tendencies and difficulties in holding down relationships, they are not joined up and rarely supported by public health initiatives,' explains Silver. There should be, she says, 'a public health response and for this to be seen as a public health crisis.'

She is disappointed by the failure of the recently published House of Commons Online Safety bill to regulate manufacturers. 'It's been lauded by the British Government as ground-breaking because Ofcom will regulate online content for the first time, but it only focuses on user-generated content. So it's great, for instance, for preventing the kind of online racial abuse which took place in the aftermath of the Euros, but there is nothing about regulating games manufacturers who need to be accountable just as the tobacco and gambling companies are.'

Silver is realistic that gaming is here to stay. 'I don't want to be a killjoy and we can't put the genie back in the lamp,

Computer game addiction: the warning signs

For most children, gaming won't become an addiction – but for a small fraction, it can. Here are the warning signs.

Obsessive behaviour

'By obsession, we mean the child will play video games and play it more at the detriment of other things around their lives falling down around them,' says Dr Joanne Orlando of Western Sydney University. If their school work or health declines, or they're losing friends to video games, that's a warning sign. '[Look for] a real and increasing obsession.'

When it's more than a phase

Squabbling over the controller isn't a cause for concern – it happens. Gaming addiction requires such behaviour to extend over 12 months. But that doesn't mean waiting a year without doing anything. Parents sensing addiction rise over that time should step in and talk to their child. Keep a diary of your observations which will be very useful if you decide to refer your child.

Get a second opinion

You may be convinced of addiction and but your doctor says otherwise. But gaming addiction is new and not always understood. 'Your local doctor won't necessarily know how to help you, nor would every single psychologist,' says Orlando. Seeking out someone who knows their stuff is vital.

Rule out other issues

Gaming addiction may not be the root cause of a child playing games. 'If parents are worried, it might also be important to consider what else is happening in the child's life at the time,' says Orlando. A sad event or major health condition can be a trigger for children to escape into video games, and some parents report the games can be a force for good in these circumstances.

especially after lockdown when it fulfilled a social need and parents found it harder to impose limits – but I was lucky.

'Aron has stopped gaming. It wasn't as a result of anything I did – although I tried.

'It happened in the past year or so as he went into sixth form. In spite of all the uncertainties of lockdown, something made him decide to focus more on his work and spend less time in the virtual world, but many others will not be as fortunate,' says Silver.

She is not wrong. It's time all of us woke up to the 'opioid' possibility of gaming, before teenage screen addiction becomes another global pandemic.

3 August 2021

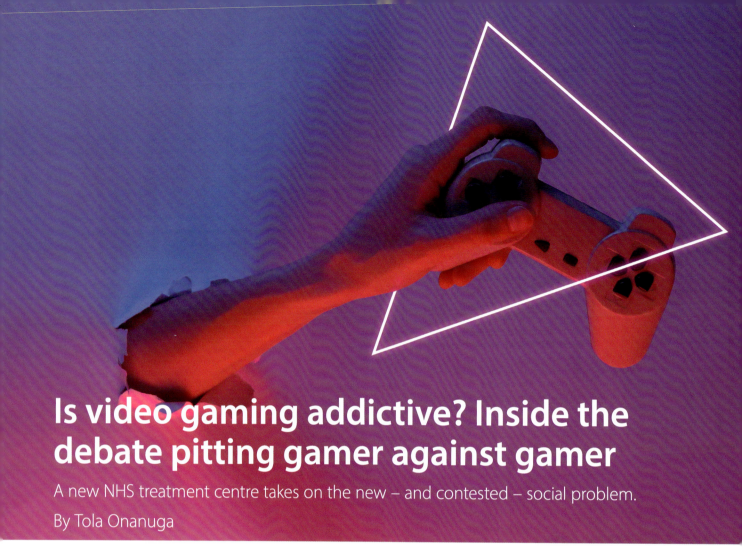

Is video gaming addictive? Inside the debate pitting gamer against gamer

A new NHS treatment centre takes on the new – and contested – social problem.

By Tola Onanuga

The first specialist NHS clinic to treat gaming addiction in the UK will open at the start of November in London, allowing children and adults who are seriously addicted to computer games to access free treatment and support, according to NHS England.

The move comes at a time when the gaming industry has experienced enormous growth over the past decade. Recent figures show that there are approximately 2.2 billion gamers across the world and the global video games industry is worth about £110 billion, a number that is estimated to rise to £140 billion by the end of 2021.

Multiplayer games such as Fortnite, released in 2017, have become a genuine pop-culture phenomenon. However, their enduring popularity among younger players, has sparked concerns about the amount of time gamers spend playing. Reports of extreme gaming addictions have risen; one horrifying case resulted in a US woman being jailed in 2011 for allowing her toddler daughter to die of malnutrition while she spent hours playing World of Warcraft, another hugely popular online multiplayer game.

More recently, a group of Canadian parents have issued a lawsuit against makers of Fortnite for allegedly making the game as addictive as cocaine and 'ruining children's lives'.

A problem or a hobby?

There is, however, much disagreement around gaming addiction, or 'gaming disorder', as it has been termed by the World Health Organization (WHO), which categorised it as a

health condition last year. The official definition states that the disorder is a pattern of persistent or recurrent gaming behaviour in which people lose control of their gaming behaviour, among other things.

This definition has prompted both praise and criticism. James Good, a gamer who formerly suffered from addiction, told Sky News that these changes will help people get the support they need. Good now works at Game Quitters, a support organisation for those 'fighting to take back their lives from video game addiction.' Conversely, director of research at the Oxford Internet Institute Andrew Przybylski has insisted that gaming addiction is 'absolutely not an addiction.' The global gaming industry is firmly opposed to the WHO's categorisation and has urged the WHO to reconsider its decision. The Entertainment Software Association, the US trade association of the industry, recently stated that the decision 'trivialises real mental health issues like depression and social anxiety disorder.'

Meanwhile the NHS England has stated that psychiatrists and clinical psychologists will work with patients aged between 13-25 whose lives are being wrecked by severe or complex behavioural issues.

Pamela Roberts, addictions programme manager at Priory Hospital Woking, says gaming disorder is a complex condition. 'Addiction or internet gaming disorder is often caused by the involvement of different influences and experiences, including a person's biology, emotional resilience, relationships and environmental factors. A complex mix of biopsychosocial factors contribute to the condition of addiction,' she explains.

Roberts stresses that most people who play games do so responsibly and without significant harm: 'According to WHO, about 1-3 per cent of the gaming population of people struggle with the symptoms of gaming disorder. But, when we consider the number of gamers is over 2 billion people, this means there are millions of people potentially struggling with addiction, as well as people at risk of developing addiction.'

Roberts also says it would be wrong to suggest the issue primarily affects children, since the average age of a gamer is 33 years old. If it is stigmatised as a child's problem, older people may find it harder to seek support, she adds.

Avoiding stigmisation

Some people who have struggled with an addiction to gaming don't agree that is should be classed as a medical disorder. This is true for Elina Ollila, chief experience officer at Kast.gg, an online hangout platform. 'This 'disorder' could span many hobbies and applies, arguably, to other groups of people as well,' she says. 'It would be the same for someone who is a gym bunny or sports enthusiast, for example. Where do we draw the line for other activities that people are strongly dedicated to? I would compare this to when my uncle, who is a diehard golf enthusiast, missed my wedding because he was so passionate about playing golf at the time.'

Ollila says better understanding of gaming behaviours is needed 'before we start to tar gamers with the same brush and bring unnecessary worry to parents who may not understand video games. It puts a negative connotation on the millions of people who enjoy playing games and I think there are far worse addictions to have that are yet to be categorised.'

A few years ago, Ollila became addicted to Clash of Clans, a wildly popular mobile strategy game which is estimated to generate $2.3 million from users daily. 'At that time, any game that had a very strong social component, such as massively multiplayer online role-playing games (World of Warcraft, for instance), was instantly attractive to me and at one point, the addiction got so severe that I even used three phones to play (my own and my two children's) with my colleagues and their friends from India. It took up so much of my life that I didn't realise how much time I was putting into the game,' she says.

Ollila overcame her addiction after she was recruited for a senior-level role at a gaming company and realised it was time to stop so she could focus on the new job and her family. She says scientists are treading new ground and while they may know how nicotine is addictive, for example, they can't pinpoint that same element in gamers as accurately. 'I worry that it could potentially stigmatise players and lead to more misconceptions about gamers as a whole,' she adds.

Most gamers are in control of their behaviour but those who are not may well need support to address the issue. As Roberts puts it: 'Those people who become addicted also need to be taken into consideration. Denying there's a problem at all leaves high numbers of people at risk. There is some accountability required [from gaming companies] in this case, even if the companies are not responsible for the disorder itself.'

The global gaming industry is unlikely to change its stance, however, even as the first NHS patients begin receiving treatment for addiction in the coming months and years.

24 October 2019

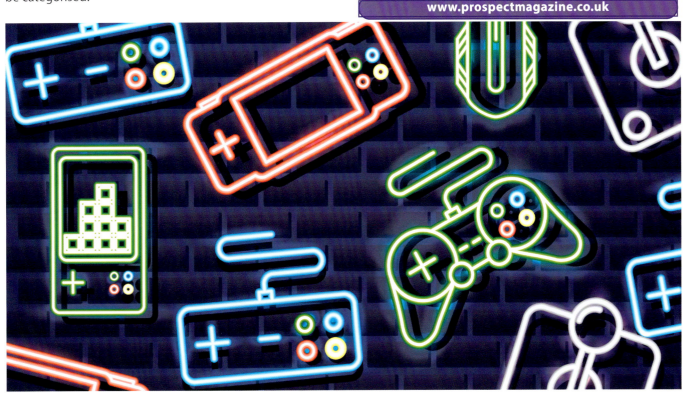

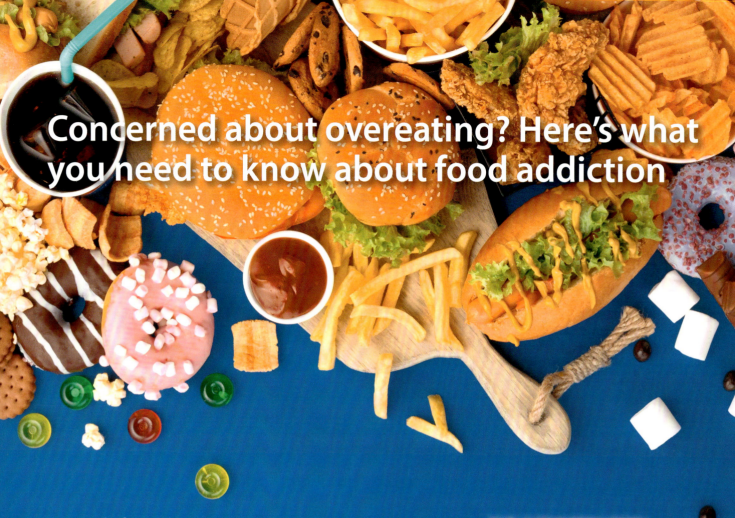

Concerned about overeating? Here's what you need to know about food addiction

An article from The Conversation.

THE CONVERSATION

By Tracy Burrows, Professor Nutrition and Dietetics, University of Newcastle & Megan Whatnall, Post-Doctoral Researcher in Nutrition and Dietetics, University of Newcastle

For many of us, eating particular foods can be comforting: a pick-me-up during a hard task; a reward after a long day at work; a satiating end to a lovely dinner.

But some people have a compulsive and uncontrolled urge to eat particular foods, especially hyper-palatable 'junk' foods. This can impact on their day-to-day functioning, and their ability to fulfil social, work or family roles.

People who struggle with addictive eating may have intense cravings, which don't relate to hunger, as well as increased levels of tolerance for large quantities of food, and feelings of withdrawal.

Rather than hunger, these cravings may be prompted by low mood, mental illness (depression and anxiety), high levels of stress, or heightened emotions.

'Food addiction' or 'addictive eating' is not yet a disorder that can be diagnosed in a clinical setting. Yet patients often ask health professionals about how to manage their addictive eating.

These health providers generally acknowledge their patients' addictive eating behaviours but may be unsure of suitable treatments.

Food addiction is commonly assessed using the Yale Food Addiction Scale.

The science of addictive eating is still emerging, but researchers are increasingly noting addiction and reward pathways in the brain triggered by stress, heightened emotions and mental illness are associated with the urge to overeat.

How common is it?

Many factors contribute to overeating. The abundance of fast food, junk food advertising, and the highly palatable ingredients of many processed foods can prompt us to eat whether we are hungry or not.

However, some people report a lack of control over their eating, beyond liking and wanting, and are seeking help for this.

Around one in six people (15-20%) report addictive patterns of eating or addictive behaviours around food.

While food addiction is higher among people with obesity and mental health conditions, it only affects a subset of these groups.

How can you tell if you have a problem?

Typically, food addiction occurs with foods that are highly palatable, processed, and high in combinations of energy, fat, salt and/or sugar while being low in nutritional value. This might include chocolates, confectionery, takeaway foods, and baked products.

These foods may be associated with high levels of reward and may therefore preoccupy your thoughts. They might elevate your mood or provide a distraction from anxious or traumatic thoughts, and over time, you may need to eat more to get the same feelings of reward.

However, for others, it could be an addiction to feelings of fullness or a sense of reward or satisfaction.

There is ongoing debate about whether it is components of food that are addictive or the behaviour of eating itself that is addictive, or a combination of the two.

Given people consume foods for a wide range of reasons, and people can form habits around particular foods, it could be different for different people.

It often starts in childhood

Through our research exploring the experiences of adults, we found many people with addictive eating attribute their behaviours to experiences that occurred in childhood.

These events are highly varied. They range from traumatic events, to the use of dieting or restrictive eating practices, or are related to poor body image or body dissatisfaction.

Our latest research found addictive eating in teenage years is associated with poorer quality of life and lower self-esteem, and it appears to increase in severity over time.

Children and adolescents tend to have fewer addictive eating behaviours, or symptoms, than adults. Of the 11 symptoms of the Yale Food Addiction Scale, children and adolescents generally have only two or three, while adults often have six or more, which is classified as severe food addiction.

The associations we observed in adolescents are also seen in adults: increased weight and poorer mental health is associated with a greater number of symptoms and prevalence of food addiction.

This highlights that some adolescents will need mental health, eating disorder and obesity services, in a combined treatment approach.

We also need to identify early risk factors to enable targeted, preventative interventions in younger age groups.

How is it treated?

The underlying causes of addictive eating are diverse so treatments can't be one-size-fits-all.

A large range of treatments are being trialled. These include:

♦ passive approaches such as self-help support groups

♦ trials of medications such as naltrexone and bupropion, which targets hormones involved in hunger and appetite and works to reduce energy intake

♦ bariatric surgery to assist with weight loss. The most common procedure in Australia is gastric banding, where an adjustable band is placed around the top part of the stomach to apply pressure and reduce appetite.

However, few of the available self-help support groups include involvement or input from qualified health professionals. While providing peer support, these may not be based on the best available evidence, with few evaluated for effectiveness.

Medications and bariatric surgery do involve health professional input and have been shown to be effective in achieving weight loss and reducing symptoms of food addiction in some people.

However, these may not be suitable for some people, such as those in the healthy weight range or with complex underlying health conditions. It's also critical people receiving medications and surgery are counselled to make diet and other lifestyle changes.

Other holistic, personalised lifestyle approaches that include diet, physical activity, as well as mindfulness, show promising results, especially when co-designed with consumers and health professionals.

Our emerging treatment program

We're also creating new holistic approaches to manage addictive eating. We recently trialled an online intervention tailored to individuals' personalities.

Delivered by dietitians and based on behaviour change research, participants in the trial received personalised feedback about their symptoms of addictive eating, diet, physical activity and sleep, and formulated goals, distraction lists, and plans for mindfulness, contributing to an overall action plan.

After three months, participants reported the program as acceptable and feasible. The next step in our research is to trial the treatment for effectiveness. We're conducting a research trial to determine the effectiveness of the treatment on decreasing symptoms of food addiction and improving mental health.

This is the first study of its kind and if found to be effective will be translated to clinical practice.

If you feel you experience addictive eating, talk to your GP.

24 November 2021

Fact or fiction – is sugar addictive?

An article from The Conversation.

THE CONVERSATION

By Amy Reichelt, Lecturer, ARC DECRA, RMIT University

Some of us can definitely say we have a sweet tooth. Whether it's cakes, chocolates, cookies, lollies or soft drinks, our world is filled with intensely pleasurable sweet treats. Sometimes eating these foods is just too hard to resist.

As a nation, Australians consume, on average, 60 grams (14 teaspoons) of table sugar (sucrose) a day. Excessive consumption of sugar is a major contributor to the increasing rates of obesity in both Australia and globally.

Eating sugary foods can become ingrained into our lifestyles and routines. That spoonful of sugar makes your coffee taste better and dessert can feel like the best part of dinner. If you've ever tried to cut back on sugar, you may have realised how incredibly difficult it is. For some people it may seem downright impossible. This leads to the question: can you be addicted to sugar?

Sugar activates the brain's reward system

Sweet foods are highly desirable due the powerful impact sugar has on the reward system in the brain called the mesolimbic dopamine system. The neurotransmitter dopamine is released by neurons in this system in response to a rewarding event.

Drugs such as cocaine, amphetamines and nicotine hijack this brain system. Activation of this system leads to intense feelings of reward that can result in cravings and addiction. So drugs and sugar both activate the same reward system in the brain, causing the release of dopamine.

This chemical circuit is activated by natural rewards and behaviours that are essential to continuing the species, such as eating tasty, high energy foods, having sex and interacting socially. Activating this system makes you want to carry out the behaviour again, as it feels good.

The criteria for substance use disorders by the Diagnostic and Statistical Manual of Mental Disorders (DSM 5) cites a variety of problems that arise when addicted to a substance. This includes craving, continuing use despite negative consequences, trying to quit but not managing to, tolerance and withdrawal. Although sugary foods are easily available, excessive consumption can lead to a number of problems similar to that of addiction. So it appears sugar may have addictive qualities. There is no concrete evidence that links sugar with an addiction/withdrawal system in humans currently, but studies using rats suggest the possibility.

Sweet attractions

Dopamine has an important role in the brain, directing our attention towards things in the environment like tasty foods that are linked to feelings of reward. The dopamine system becomes activated at the anticipation of feelings of pleasure.

This means our attention can be drawn to cakes and chocolates when we're not necessarily hungry, evoking cravings. Our routines can even cause sugar cravings. We can subconsciously want a bar of chocolate or a fizzy drink in the afternoon if this is a normal part of our daily habits.

Sugar tolerance

Repeated activation of the dopamine reward system, for example by eating lots of sugary foods, causes the brain to adapt to the frequent reward system stimulation. When we enjoy lots of these foods on a regular basis, the system starts to change to prevent it becoming overstimulated. In particular, dopamine receptors start to down-regulate.

Now there are fewer receptors for the dopamine to bind to, so the next time we eat these foods, their effect is blunted. More sugar is needed the next time we eat in order to get the same feeling of reward. This is similar to tolerance in drug addicts, and leads to escalating consumption. The negative consequences of unrestrained consumption of sugary foods include weight gain, dental cavities and developing metabolic disorders including type-2 diabetes.

Quitting sugar leads to withdrawal

Sugar can exert a powerful influence over behaviour, making cutting it out of our diets very difficult. And quitting eating a high sugar diet 'cold turkey' leads to withdrawal effects.

The length of unpleasant withdrawal symptoms following a sugar 'detox' varies. Some people quickly adjust to functioning without sugar, while others may experience severe cravings and find it very difficult to resist sugary foods.

The withdrawal symptoms are thought to be factors of individual sensitivity to sugar as well as the dopamine system readjusting to a sugar-free existence. The temporary drop in dopamine levels are thought to cause many of the psychological symptoms including cravings, particularly as our environment is filled with sweet temptations that you now have to resist.

Why quit sugar?

Cutting sugar from your diet may not be easy, as so many processed or convenience foods have added sugars hidden in their ingredients. Switching from sugar to a sweetener (Stevia, aspartame, sucralose) can cut down on calories, but it is still feeding the sweet addiction. Similarly, sugar 'replacements' like agave, rice syrup, honey and fructose are just sugar in disguise, and activate the brain's reward system just as readily as sucrose.

Physically, quitting sugar in your diet can help with weight loss, may reduce acne, improve sleep and moods, and could stop those 3pm slumps at work and school. And if you do reduce sugar consumption, sugary foods that were previously eaten to excess can taste overpoweringly sweet due to a recalibration of your sweetness sensation, enough to discourage over-consumption!

22 February 2017

The Sugar Challenge: how to kick your addiction to the white stuff and lose weight

Sugar consumption has soared during lockdown, but much of it is hidden in foods that aren't obviously sweet – here's how to cut down.

By Lauren Libbert

If there's one thing we can do to improve our health as we emerge from this pandemic, it is to eat less sugar. Comfort eating has soared as coronavirus has swept through the nation, with the latest National Diet and Nutrition Survey showing the average adult is eating roughly 12 teaspoons of sugar a day, double the recommended amount.

Manufacturers have capitalised on the need for a sweet kick in tough times. Krispy Kreme in the USA announced this week that is offering a free doughnut to anyone who gets the vaccine, and Irn-Bru has rolled out a nostalgic spin-off drink based on an old recipe, Irn-Bru 1901, which contains even more sugar than the original.

Even if you think of yourself as a healthy eater who doesn't consume too much of the white stuff, if your diet includes bread, snacks, cereals, yoghurts, gravy granules and jars of sauces – anything packaged and that comes out of a factory, basically – then chances are you do.

The Government recommends that free sugars – those added to food or drinks, as well as sugars found naturally in honey, syrups and unsweetened fruit and vegetable juices, smoothies and purées – should not make up more than 5 per cent of the energy you get from food and drink a day and adults should have no more than 30g of sugar daily.

Yet the National Diet and Nutrition Survey published in December 2020, shows adults are exceeding this recommendation by almost double with our intake of free sugars at 9.9 per cent of energy intake.

'It's very easy to eat your 30g or six teaspoons of sugar before you've even left the house in the morning,' says Sarah Flower, nutritionist and author of 22 books including Eating to Beat Type 2 Diabetes and The Sugar-Free Family Cookbook. 'Breakfast cereals, toast and jam, cereal bars, low-fat yoghurts, fruit juices, smoothies – they all add up.'

Many scientists believe added sugar is the main culprit in the obesity epidemic and the lack of Government regulation around it.

'It's all well and good to say that we shouldn't have more than 30g a day,' says Holly Gabriel, nutrition manager at charity Action on Sugar. 'But you can buy a coffee from somewhere like Starbucks, for example, which will have double that amount of sugar in it and the lack of labelling or transparency means you don't even know.'

The truth is there's no nutritional need for sugar at all. 'It doesn't contain any nutrients, but it can be very detrimental to our health, creating an insulin-resistant profile and inflammatory body, which is linked to type 2 diabetes, obesity, heart disease and more,' says Flower.

'Sugar – or glucose to be precise – is harmful in our bloodstream so our pancreas secretes the hormone insulin, which transports the glucose to be stored as glycogen in our liver or muscles. However, with our western diet, our natural stores in our liver and muscle are already full to capacity, which means we have to push the glucose into our cells to be stored as fat. High insulin levels not only mean a larger waistline but have very serious implications for our overall health.'

The fridge/freezer analogy favoured by Dr Jason Fung, a Canadian nephrologist and leading expert on intermittent fasting and low carb diets for treating type 2 diabetes, is a useful explanation. Fung explains that if you buy groceries, you first store them in the fridge. Once the fridge is full, you then store them in the freezer. Only when the food in the fridge is gone do you want to go downstairs to that cold dank basement to get the food in the freezer. 'If you're always consuming sugar your glycogen 'fridge' is full and you won't use any of your fat in the 'freezer',' says Flower.

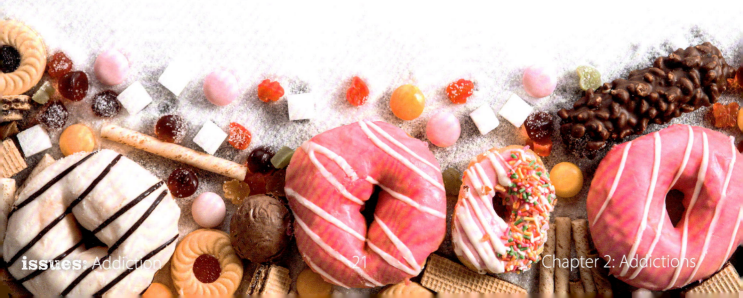

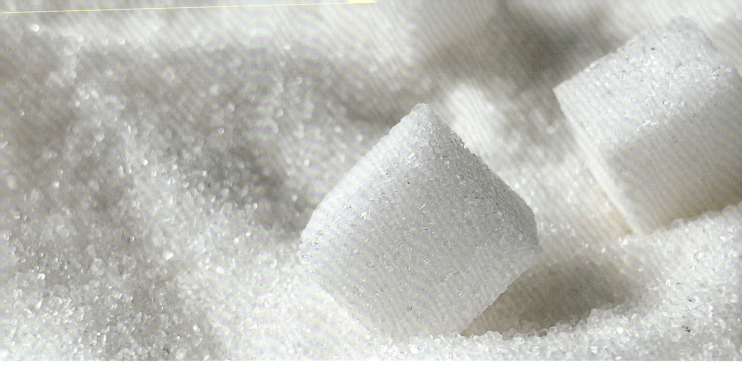

For those who argue that sugar is a natural food found in fruits in the form of fructose – and therefore must be good for you – there is an important distinction to make.

'Eating a whole fruit means you're also eating some fibre, which slows the digestion of the fructose and the rate at which it enters your bloodstream so that's always the best way to eat fruit,' says Flower.

But the fructose found in ultra-processed foods in the form of high fructose corn syrups and fruit concentrates has much – or all – of the fibre and nutrients removed.

'Processed fructose is now deemed to be the most damaging sugar form and is linked to non-alcoholic fatty liver disease (NAFLD) and heart disease,' adds Flower.

Fructose also interferes with our leptin response, which is our body's natural appetite suppressant. When the brain stops getting the message to stop eating, it leads to the laying down of more visceral fat around your vital organs.

But coming off the white stuff can be tricky if you do a sudden cold turkey. Research shows sugar can also be addictive, triggering dopamine 'hits' in the brain, and can create changes in the brain similar to those found in people who are addicted to cocaine and alcohol.

'After having something sugary, we get a lovely sugar rush, increasing our energy and the feelgood factor all at once plus stimulating the craving hormone, ghrelin, that nags at us to eat more and more,' says Flower. 'The bad news is we then crash within a few hours to have much lower blood sugar, leaving us feeling tired, and again wanting more.'

The key when starting to think about cutting sugar from your diet is to look at food labels. Gabriel points out that there are many names that manufacturers use for sugar to hide them from us. Some of these include agave syrup, honey, molasses, rice syrup, corn syrup, maltose, crystallised fructose and so on. 'The higher up the ingredient list, the more is in there but look out for these different types of sugars too on the label as they might not be instantly recognisable.'

Gabriel also warns against foods that have 'health halos': considered healthy but actually aren't. 'Take granola bars,'

she says. 'Just because something states it is sugar-free does not mean it is sugar-free. It can simply mean they haven't added sugar but they can sweeten with a whole host of other sugars such as dates, syrups and honey or it can contain dried fruit, which has been completely macerated.'

Trainer and nutritionist Harley Pasternak co-founded Sweetkick, a mint that temporarily suppresses the taste of sweetness and knows far too well how challenging kicking sugar can be.

'We are consuming three to four times the amount of sugar we should safely be consuming and if you want to reduce the amount you eat, you have to start with a food log, knowing how much you're actually eating and what sugars are your weakness, then minimise the presence of these foods in your home and do a high sugar purge in your kitchen,' says Pasternak. 'Next, focus on what you should be eating, rather than what you shouldn't be eating. Every meal should have protein, fibre and healthy fats to ensure your blood sugar is stable.'

Gabriel agrees. 'Sugar doesn't give you any feeling of satiety at all and you can eat a huge amount and still feel hungry,' she says. 'But proteins like chicken, lean red meat, beans, pulses, eggs and healthy fats such as avocados, nuts and seeds will fill you up more so you'll end up eating far less sugar.'

Cutting sugar out of your diet isn't easy. A good first step is to take our 7-day Sugar Challenge, which gives you one strategy a day for reducing your sugar intake. 'I don't believe you need to completely cut sugar from your diet,' says Pasternak. 'You just need to reduce the amount of sugar you're consuming. A little bit of sugar is OK. A lot is not good.' With that in mind, take one day at a time and watch as you start to feel more energetic and more focused and may even lose a little weight.

26 March 2021

Caffeine

What is caffeine?

Caffeine is a drug that is found in tea, coffee, cocoa, many soft drinks such as colas and some chocolates. It is also used in a wide variety of medicines especially cold remedies.

Caffeine can be manufactured in a laboratory but it mainly comes from the Arabian coffee shrub, commercial tea plants, cocoa beans and kola nuts. Coffee is grown in many areas of the world including Africa, Arabia, Central and South America, Java and Sumatra and the West Indies. Tea is mainly grown in eastern Asia and South America especially India, China, Indonesia, Sri Lanka and Japan. Most of the world's cocoa is grown in West Africa.

On average in the UK, we drink nearly 100 million cups of tea per day, each cup containing about 40mg of caffeine, but more if the tea is left to brew longer.

Coffee is almost as popular with 95 million cups of coffee consumed a day. About 80% of coffee drunk at home is instant coffee containing around 60mg of caffeine per cup.

History

Tea and cocoa have been drunk for thousands of years. Earliest use of tea was coffee probably in China before the 10th century BC. Coffee use is much more recent and the first record of its cultivation was in Arabia about 675 AD. Tea was first imported to Europe in about 1600 by the Dutch East India Company and first came to the UK in about 1660.

Coffee was first introduced to the UK as a medicine but became very fashionable to drink in the 1670s. Coffee houses sprang up in London. They attracted literary figures such as Hogarth and Swift, political revolutionaries and financial entrepreneurs – some of the first banks and the Stock Exchange were started in coffee houses. Coffee houses caused much controversy. The authorities saw them as recruiting places for political radicals and women's groups protested that they damaged family life. The authorities moved to close down all the coffee houses in London. A compromise was reached where coffee houses could remain open so long as they did not allow the sale of political books and pamphlets or political speeches.

Coffee houses became less popular and changes in commerce saw coffee consumption fall. England turned to tea drinking and remains the only country in Europe that consumes more tea than coffee. In recent years concerns about the effects of caffeine have led to the manufacture of decaffeinated coffees and teas.

The law

There are no legal restrictions on the sale or use of coffee, tea, cocoa, soft drinks and chocolate confectionery. Certain medicines which contain caffeine may only be available on a doctor's prescription.

Effects/risks

Caffeine is an 'upper' and helps stimulate the body, increasing heart rate and blood pressure. It combats tiredness and drowsiness and makes people feel more alert and able to concentrate. Many people have a cup of tea or coffee every morning to 'get going'. However, people also drink tea and coffee to help them relax. Caffeine also makes people urinate more. High doses can result in people having headaches and feeling very irritable.

People who drink more than 6 to 8 cups of normal strength tea or coffee a day usually become dependent.

They may find it difficult to stop using and experience withdrawal symptoms if they try. This can include feeling tired and anxious and suffering headaches.

'I don't know if I could do without coffee. That first cup in the morning gets me up. Off to work and the first thing is coffee. Basically I drink at least 8 cups a day and the stronger the better. If you said to me don't drink coffee tomorrow I would get very anxious about trying to do it. I don't think I would last very long without it.'

Research into the health effects of long term use of caffeine is inconclusive. However, some reports have suggested that it can lead to a higher incidence of asthma, peptic ulcers, kidney, bladder and heart disease and blood pressure problems.

'We have seen several well-marked cases of coffee excess... The sufferer is tremulous, and looses his self-command; he is subject to fits of agitation and depression; he looses colour and has a haggard appearance. The appetite falls off, and symptoms of gastric catarrh may be manifested. The heart also suffers; it palpitates, or it intermits. As with other such agents, a renewed dose of the poison gives temporary relief, but at the cost of future misery'. Sir T.C. Allbutt and H.D. Rolleston A system of medicine 1909.

There have also been concerns about the amount of caffeine consumed by young children particularly in soft drinks and chocolate. Some commentators have suggested that children who consume a lot of caffeine may become hyperactive. A child drinking one can of cola will be taking the equivalent caffeine intake as an adult drinking four cups of coffee.

April 2022

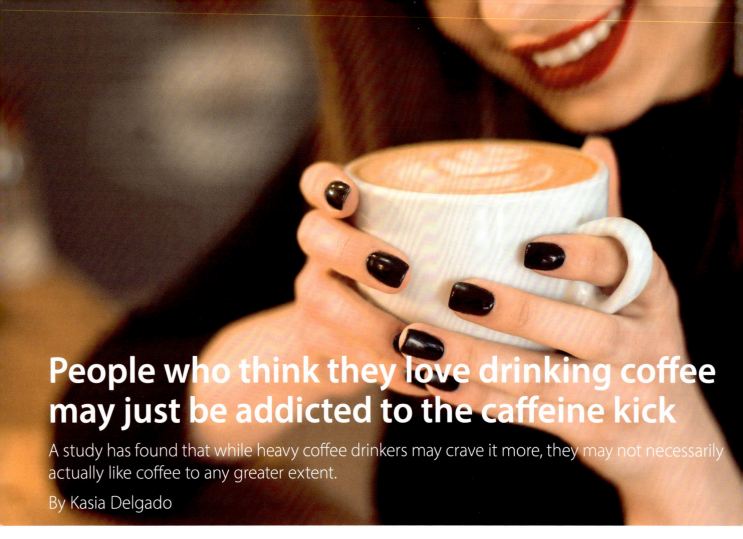

People who think they love drinking coffee may just be addicted to the caffeine kick

A study has found that while heavy coffee drinkers may crave it more, they may not necessarily actually like coffee to any greater extent.

By Kasia Delgado

Coffee drinkers come in various forms. There are those who down a cup of instant once a day just to wake up, and then there are those who grind their own beans and take an interest in which dark roast from Colombia has notes of blackberry and chocolate.

We all know someone – or perhaps we are someone – in the latter camp, who loves coffee like a hobby. It's part of their identity; if they were in the market for a partner, it's the sort of thing they'd put on their Tinder profile. They drink the stuff until nightfall, and will slip out of a meeting or away from their family on holiday to hunt down the best flat white in town. They just love the taste.

However, a study has found that while heavy coffee drinkers may crave it more, they may not necessarily actually like coffee to any greater extent.

Nicolas Koranyi at the University of Jena, Germany, and colleagues found that heavy coffee drinkers want coffee a lot more than they like it. The implication is that they drink it mostly or entirely to feed their addiction, rather than for pleasure. 'Addiction can be characterised as a condition where increases in wanting are not met by concurrent increases in liking,' says Koranyi.

Craving coffee

Caffeine is likely to have a much weaker effect on this system than other addictive drugs, but the study suggests that the way the brain engages with it is similar. The results of a psychological test on 56 students revealed that heavy coffee drinkers had a strong wanting for coffee – much more than the light drinkers. But both heavy and light drinkers showed a similarly low liking for coffee.

However coffee is a vital part of many people's routines, in part because of the energy boost it can provide, but also because of the way it is marketed as an experience. In the 90s, 'coffees became more personal, more accessible,' says anthropologist and Scientific American Krystal D'Costa. 'The group that the market feared it had lost, the 20 to 29-year-olds, had been netted. People began to drink coffee because it meant something to them: a flavour for everyone, a style for every lifestyle – we have methodically been taught to socialise over coffee, to look for a boost in productivity.'

However, does the new study mean that a self-confessed coffee lover, for whom coffee is part of their identity, is simply addicted to the stuff? Yes, perhaps, but it depends on the person.

Someone who drinks, say, two cups a day is not a 'heavy user', will still have a mild addiction, but can also like the stuff too.

It's just that someone who doesn't really like coffee can still want it because their brain has come to rely on that caffeine kick. Either way, sit back and enjoy that cappuccino; you'll at least think you're loving it.

8 December 2020

Teenagers fell in love with energy drinks years ago, but now parents see the harmful effects

Evidence is growing that the caffeinated, sugary drinks are harmful to children's wellbeing.

By Susie Mesure

For many teenagers, energy drinks offer a cheap buzz, an instant early-morning boost when they need to be at school but would rather be in bed. Better still, are those such as G Fuel that promise the elixir of endurance and enhanced focus for virtual battles into the early hours.

Little wonder that up to one third of UK children, mostly young teens, consume at least one energy drink a week, with some reaching for one almost daily, according to a Government-funded study published in BMJ Open.

Formulations vary but the drinks all come loaded with caffeine and often sugar, providing a palatable alternative to a simple cup of coffee. And all for as little as 50p for a can of Bulldog Power, a Dutch drink that pledges to deliver 'British Spirit', at your local corner store, or at least at mine in south London. (Several supermarkets refuse to sell the drinks to under-16s.)

Why fret about possible headaches and being too wired to sleep when that doesn't seem to bother the TikTok influencers pushing brands such as G Fuel on thirsty gamers?

And yet, researchers worry these drinks just aren't very good for under 18s – children, in other words. That's why UK Government has said it will ban sales to children, because advice and warning labels are not cutting through, although the ban – when it eventually arrives – will only affect under-16s.

Research by Mintel, based on a lifestyle survey in April 2021, suggests teenagers are the main consumers of the drinks: 54 per cent of 16- to 19-year-olds drink energy drinks, compared with an average of 31 per cent of Britons overall. This is despite worrying about the negative effects: 66 per cent of those teenagers were concerned they had trouble sleeping.

Claire Khouja of the University of York, lead researcher on the study, said researchers had found consistent evidence of links between regularly consuming energy drinks and harmful effects on children's overall wellbeing. She added: 'These findings offer support for a government policy banning the sale of energy drinks to children.'

The latest study, commissioned by the Department of Health and Social Care, analysed data on thousands of UK children, as well as consumption by youngsters in other countries from around the world, including the US and Canada. Because the findings rely on surveys, the researchers stress they cannot prove that energy drinks cause problems for children.

Energy drink makers have had teenagers in their sights ever since the likes of Red Bull bounded into the UK market in 1997. That summer, stalls piled with free cans of the original medicinal-flavoured concoction were a staple of student parties and balls in universities.

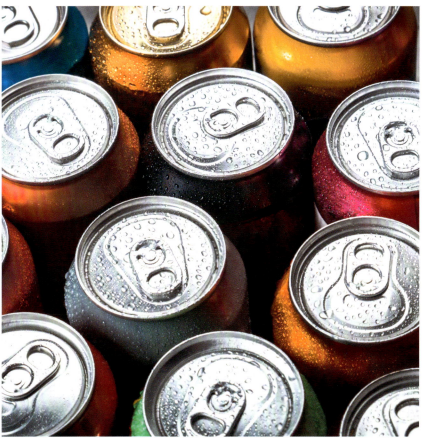

These days it's even easier to tempt teens thanks to YouTube and TikTok. Claire Morton, a life coach and meditation teacher who runs her own business, The Purpose Pusher Project, says her 13-year-old son has been drinking energy drinks for two years. 'He got into them because they were advertised to give you better focus and better concentration on your PC games, which I thought was a little bit naughty,' she says.

Morton, who is from Liverpool, is trying to avoid banning her son from drinking them. 'I'd rather educate him. I tell him, "everything in moderation but water is best",' she tells me. He used to have an energy drink with breakfast, claiming it helped him to concentrate, but now waits until after school.

She tries keeping tabs on how many he drinks but admits it can be as many as three or four a day. 'They can change his moods and make him a little bit hyper. It's hard keeping an eye on him. I know some of his friends drink a lot more,' she adds.

Abbie Chadd, director of A Level Revision UK, is among those who wish they wouldn't. She singles out male students as the worst culprits, something the researchers also found from the global datasets they studied. 'I haven't seen any benefits,' she tells i.

'[Energy drinks] may make children alert in the short term but they are essentially a form of stimulant so there is a comedown,' says Chadd. 'More often than not, students who have consumed these drinks will start to lack concentration and will often become agitated and distracted especially if required to concentrate for sustained periods of time.'

Research based on surveys cannot prove that energy drinks cause problems for children. 'It's difficult to establish cause and effect,' adds Khouja. But definitive data on the ill effects of the ingredients in energy drinks, from caffeine to stimulants such as guanine and taurine, is scarce because it would be unethical to get kids overdosing in a laboratory.

But there is plenty of anecdotal evidence that excessive consumption is harmful. One sixth-form teacher, who works at a boys' grammar school, says: 'Pupils drink energy drinks plus espresso in the morning to get them going. A lot of teenage boys really struggle to get up early enough for school. This is unfortunately how quite a few of my older students manage. I had one Year 13 boy last year who physically shook in our morning registration.'

Helena Gibson-Moore, nutrition scientist, at the British Nutrition Foundation, says the trouble with relying on energy drinks for a boost is that most contain large doses of caffeine and sugar. Some also contain ingredients like guarana, another form of caffeine. A 500ml can of energy drink can contain 20 teaspoons of sugar and the same amount of caffeine as two cups of coffee.

'Regular use of energy drinks has been linked to headaches, sleeping problems, anxiety and behavioural changes, likely caused by caffeine. The sugar content may also contribute to calorie intakes and increase the risk of tooth decay,' says Gibson-Moore.

Various health organisations around the world, including the American Academy of Paediatrics, recommend that energy drinks are not appropriate for teenagers. In the UK the Food Standards Agency advises that children should only consume caffeine in moderation, and healthy eating advice from the Department of Health and Social care states that caffeinated drinks are unsuitable for toddlers and young children.

The British Soft Drinks Association is adamant its members do not market or promote energy drinks to under 16s. 'Nor do they sample products with this age group,' says Gavin Partington, the group's director general. 'We remain committed to supporting the responsible sale of energy drinks.'

18 February 2022

Doctors call for energy drinks ban for under-18s

Links to harmful behaviour and concerns over addiction have prompted doctors to call for a ban on the sale of energy drinks to under-18s in Scotland.

The Royal College of Physicians of Edinburgh (RCPE) says research in recent years into the impact of the caffeine-laden drinks has found association with sensation seeking behaviour, binge drinking, smoking and a greater risk of depression and injuries.

The Scottish government is currently consulting on whether restrictions should be introduced to prevent energy drinks being sold to children under 16.

In its response, the RCPE suggests the age limit should be set to a higher limit of 18-years-old, in line with legislation on the purchase of tobacco and alcohol.

It has also suggested an end to the sale of energy drinks from vending machines, as it would be difficult to enforce age restrictions.

The RCPE response said: 'Age verification processes already exist for the sale of other restricted products (tobacco and alcohol) to the young.

'A ban on the sales of energy drinks for young people under the age of 18 would be the most practical and easiest to implement for retailers building on these processes.

'The introduction of mandatory age restrictions… is necessary to create a consistent approach across all retailers while protecting the health of our young people.'

Last year hospitals and all publicly-funded sports centres in Scotland banned the sale of energy drinks to children aged under 16.

The RCPE added: 'Public health information campaigns in schools as well as in the general public would help support a change in behaviour and reduce excess consumption of energy drinks by children, particularly in the home.'

6 March 2020

Energy drinks and young people

By Dr Bunmi Aboaba, Creator of the Food Addiction Coach Accelerator Program

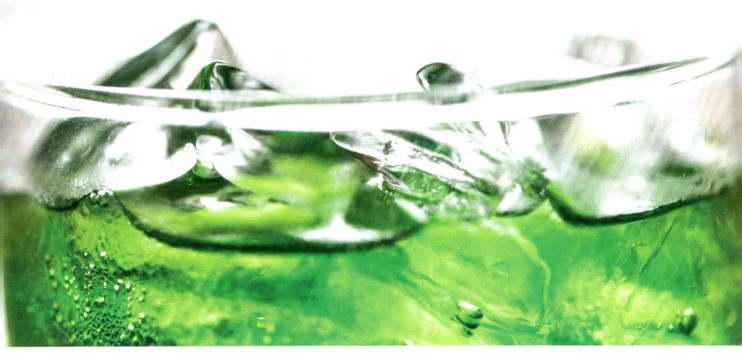

Energy drinks are hugely popular among young people, with an estimated 50% of weekly consumption coming from children and teenagers. Last year, the energy drink industry was valued at $61 billion, with a future projection of $100 billion by 2027. However, regular consumption is linked to serious health effects.

It is vital that children and young people have a balanced and nutritious diet, as well as enjoying regular physical activity, in order to flourish mentally, physically and socially. The importance of diet and exercise for young people's mental and physical health will be no surprise to those working in the physical activity sector, however, I want to highlight in particular the negative consequences caused by regular consumption of energy drinks.

Inside energy drinks

Energy drinks are marketed as a means to increase alertness, stamina, and energy levels. These drinks are often aggressively marketed towards adolescents to increase sports prowess, concentration when studying, and boost energy if tired.

Some beverages purport to include vitamins, herbs and nutrients such as ginseng, guarana, and taurine. However, the two most significant ingredients are caffeine and sugar. The majority contain approximately 200mg of caffeine – around two cups of strong coffee – and equal sugar to a can of fizzy drink.

There is a severe lack of regulation towards the ingredients of these beverages, as caffeine, sugar, guarana, and taurine are all 'active' ingredients which can cause harm. For example:

♦ Caffeine – Increased anxiety, elevated blood pressure, cardiovascular issues and the risk of seizure and heart failure.

♦ Sugar – Stress, dental issues, obesity, and type two diabetes.

♦ Vitamin B – Skin conditions, liver toxicity, blurred vision and nerve damage.

♦ Stimulants including guarana and taurine – sleep problems, anxiety, restlessness, upset stomach, and quickened heartbeat.

Numerous studies show an association between regular consumption of these drinks and various adverse health effects, including:

♦ Stress

♦ Aggression

♦ High blood pressure

♦ Increased obesity

♦ Type 2 diabetes

♦ Poor sleep

♦ Nausea and stomach irritation

♦ Headaches and eye strain

♦ Dental erosion

♦ Mental health issues.

Caffeine overdose

Some energy drinks contain as much as 500mg, equivalent to fourteen cans of cola.

The American Academy of Paediatrics recommends a daily limit of less than 100mg of caffeine for young people aged 12 to 18-years-old. There is no recommended safe limit for children under the age of 12.

Caffeine and other stimulants can cause dangerous changes in heart function and blood pressure, as it stimulates the release of norepinephrine. Norepinephrine is a stress hormone which increases heart rate.

Consuming too much caffeine can cause a caffeine overdose. More than approximately 150-200mg of caffeine per kilogram of body weight is considered lethal. Overdosing on caffeine can cause vomiting, palpitations, high blood pressure, seizures and, potentially, fatality.

The amount consumed to trigger overdose varies, with children and teenagers more susceptible than adults. In 2017, a 16-year-old boy from South Carolina in America, died from a caffeine overdose which triggered a heart arrhythmia after drinking one soda, one latte and an energy drink. Greater education and legislation around energy drinks can help to avoid future cases of caffeine overdose and protect the lives of young people.

Mental health

An important study published earlier this year evidenced the adverse mental health effects of regular energy drink consumption on young people. The study demonstrated that children and teenagers who drank energy drinks each week were likely to have decreased overall wellbeing.

Evidence demonstrated consistent associations between energy drinks and:

- Anxiety and depression
- Self-harm and suicide
- Hyperactivity
- Decreased academic performance
- Headaches
- Irritability and aggression
- Alcohol use and smoking
- Sleep problems

This study found that boys are more likely to consume greater quantities of energy drinks than girls, as were those from lower socio-economic groups.

Healthy alternatives

Encourage your children and teenagers to try one of the below healthy alternatives the next time they are looking for a natural boost:

- Smoothies – fruit and vegetable smoothies are an excellent choice as long as you do not add extra sugars. Berries, citrus, spinach, kale, and parsley are particularly good at boosting energy levels and providing your body and brain with essential vitamins.

- Green tea – for those over the age of 12, green tea can provide many health benefits. Green tea is widely reported to have numerous positive effects on metabolism, heart function, and the brain, and still contains 25-40mg of caffeine.

- Coconut water – packed full of potassium, magnesium, phosphorus, and calcium, coconut water is a healthy and refreshing alternative to energy drinks.

- Water – when dehydrated, our metabolism slows down and we feel tired, drained, and sluggish. Rehydrating with water acts quickly and boosts our energy levels, improves concentration, and elevates our mood. Try adding some fresh fruit to your water for extra vitamins and minerals to provide even more energy.

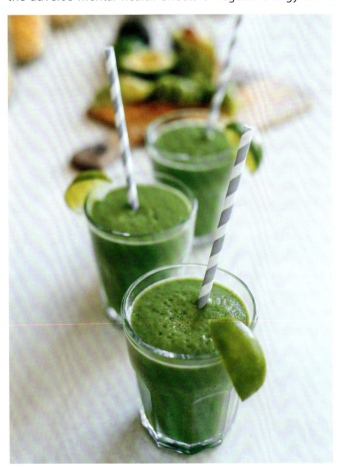

What is it like to have shopping addiction and how to deal with it

By Pamela Roberts

For those who are addicted, shopping is the medicine – usually a temporary comfort from stress, anxiety, loneliness, and fear for example, chased closely by guilt and shame. This then needs 'comforting' with more shopping 'medicine'. Addiction is a vicious cycle.

Stepping away from shopping addiction requires firstly figuring out whether you have the problem. If you honestly answer 'yes' to any of the following questions, Shopaholics Anonymous suggests you may have an addiction:

- Do you shop when you feel angry or disappointed?

- Has overspending created problems in your life?

- Do you have conflicts with loved ones about your need to shop?

- While shopping, do you feel euphoric rushes or anxiety?

- After shopping, do you feel like you have just finished doing something wild or dangerous?

- After shopping, do you ever feel ashamed, guilty or embarrassed about what you have done?

- Do you frequently buy things that you never end up using or wearing?

- Do you think about money almost all the time?

Attempts to stop shopping will cause many people addicted to shopping to experience withdrawal symptoms, not dissimilar to the withdrawals a person will have when addicted to alcohol or drugs.

It is such a surprise to learn that withdrawals are not just about a physical dependence to a substance. Psychological withdrawals are often more subtle but equally overwhelming. Of course, withdrawals vary from person to person and are often noticed as a feeling of irritability, depression.

If you know you have a problem with shopping addiction and understanding that there will be withdrawals, a next good step is getting help. It's a good idea to remove shopping apps but of course any 'good addict' knows these can simply be downloaded again. It will require determination, in your most desperate moments:

- Pay attention to your relationship with money. Sometimes this is intertwined with generational financial legacies, attitudes and experiences with money that are passed through the family line. Identifying patterns of behaviour and beliefs won't cure the addiction but it can help in understanding some of the potential underlying monetary matters

- Consider how you handled money in childhood, and the financial circumstances of the family. How was money regarded and managed? What were the influences towards money from grandparents or older generations?

- It's impossible for someone addicted to shopping to stop shopping completely, and hoarding and deprivation are

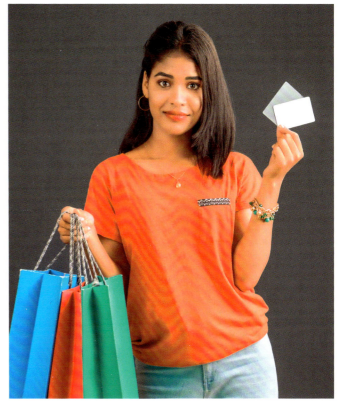

simply the other extreme. So, recovery involves starting to pay attention to finances, keep an eye on expenditure, and create a spending plan. In this way instead of indulging or depriving, a plan helps to determine what's affordable, what's necessary. It enables you to make choices rather than spend uncontrollably

- Stop using your credit card. Rather than try to do this alone (addiction, after all, is isolating), seek out some support. There are self-help groups where it's possible to find out how other people manage the need for comfort through shopping. There are also people who understand without judgement. These can often be people where you can remain honest and accountable – going underground simply keeps the need to escape alive and strong

Recovery from any addiction, including shopping addiction, is never going to be a straight line. This is a process of learning and change. It does require a change of thinking and attitude which not only takes time but also requires help. This does require active engagement with the process of change, it doesn't just happen. It's not easy; hence the self-help groups can bolster the changes especially when the temptation to shop is strong. And it will be. It's not impossible, however, to overcome this with the right help.

9 March 2021

www.psychreg.org

www.Pamela-Roberts.co.uk

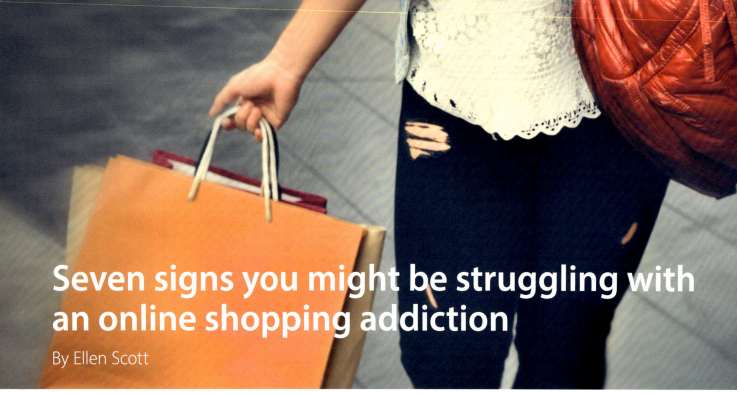

Seven signs you might be struggling with an online shopping addiction

By Ellen Scott

Now we're out of lockdown and free to leave the house again, you might have thought this was the end of your online shopping reliance.

But some habits are hard to break.

The ease of clicking, ordering, and eagerly awaiting deliveries may have allowed what started out as a convenience to develop into a full-blown online shopping addiction.

And with actual outside-the-house socialising back on the cards, we now have even more excuses to spend.

So, how can you tell when your online shopping has become a problem?

The experts at Delamere Health share seven signs that you could be struggling with a shopping addiction.

You spend hours a day scrolling through online shops

Take a serious look at your daily screentime, and track which sites and apps are soaking up the bulk of your hours.

In theory, you should only really be going on to a shopping site when you need something specific. If you spend hours 'just browsing', but more often than not find yourself buying whatever nice bits you spot, this could be an issue.

You spend more than you can afford

'This is a common issue for those suffering from an addiction,' say the team at Delamere. 'An addiction can lead to a feeling of lack of control – and this can include the amount we spend.

'Much like gambling addiction, shopping addiction can have a hugely negative impact on our finances.

'Many may find themselves dipping into their savings, remortgaging homes and even in some cases borrowing or stealing from partners/family or friends to fund their addiction.'

When your mind is operating on a logical basis, you'll have a budget and know that you simply can't go over it. When you have a shopping addiction, that knowledge gets chucked out of the window – you'll spend money you don't have just to get a fix.

You don't feel like you're in control

Ever feel like you momentarily blacked out and went on a spree? Find yourself feeling clueless about where all your money has gone at the end of the month?

Or is the opposite true – do you feel out of control in all areas of your life, apart from shopping? Does clicking 'buy' feel like a moment of peace amid chaos?

A loss of control – whether when you're online shopping or as a trigger for it – is a sign of addiction.

'For those with an addiction, repeating the unhealthy action can sometimes feel like the only way they can regain control of their lives,' explain the experts.

'With shopping addiction, placing an order is the only way some people may feel like they can feel in control for a brief period of time. It is important to try to remember that this feeling of control will fade again and breaking a cycle like this is important for our mental health.'

You get an urge to shop when you feel upset or angry

For you, there's always a reason to spend – and it's often to deal with difficult emotions.

If online shopping is your first port of call to distract yourself from feeling sad, bored, lonely, or fed up, that could signal you have an addiction.

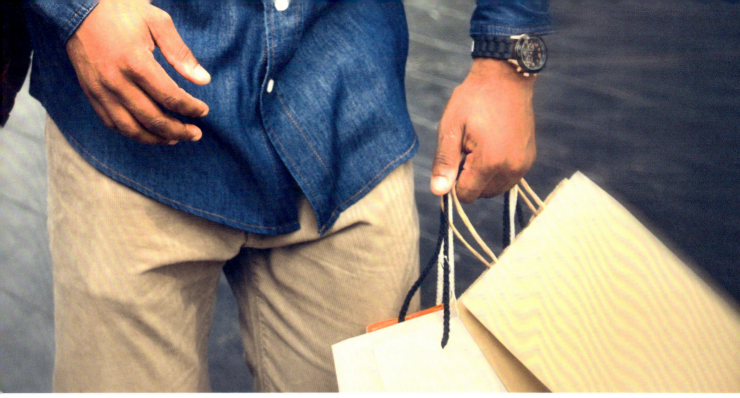

You feel a genuine 'high' when you shop

The Delamere team says: 'Do you ever get a feeling of exhilaration and/or anxiety whenever you place an order?

'We have all got excited now and again about an order – but if shopping gives you an intense rush (as if you have just been on a rollercoaster) every time, then this may be a sign of addiction.

'Euphoric rushes are caused by surges of the brain chemical dopamine. Much like a drug addiction, the brain will produce less dopamine each time as it gets used to the activity.

'However, the body then craves the exhilarating feeling and therefore people can feel like they need to increase the amount they spend, or number of orders they place, in order to get the 'highs' they are craving.'

You buy so much that you have items you've never worn or used

Take a peek through your wardrobe. Are there multiple things with tags still on, or that you really question buying?

You stay up late to shop

If your shopping habit is leaving you bleary-eyed and exhausted, that's a surefire sign that something's not right.

'Many people with addiction struggle to switch off,' the experts say. 'At night, those with an online shopping addiction can find themselves unable to sleep and reaching for their phones, and specifically their shopping apps, for comfort.

'Those with an online shopping addiction may find themselves more prone to shop on an evening or when they're in bed with nothing else to do or concentrate on.

'If you do relate to this then many can find that doing calm exercises, e.g. yoga, before bed can help relax the body. We would also recommend turning off your phone or leaving it in another room for the night so you are less tempted to reach for it.'

It's important that if you feel you are struggling with a shopping addiction, you seek proper support. Talk to your GP or therapist to discuss this further and work on treatment.

In the meantime, there are some steps you can take to reduce the urge to shop:

♦ Remove shopping apps from your phone

♦ Delete your card details from your web browser and each shop's site

♦ Monitor the amount of time you spend scrolling online

♦ Understand that it is not the norm to have the same amount of clothes and other possessions as influencers – most of these items will be sent back to brands

♦ Try the 48-hour rule. Any time you're about to buy something online, leave it for 48 hours to see if you still want or need it, or if the urge has gone

♦ Give yourself a savings goal to work towards

20 August 2020

Children of addicted parents

By Katherine Jenkins and Matt Serlin

Having someone in your life who misuses drugs or alcohol can be extremely tough on you. They might be difficult to talk to or might act in worrying or frightening ways. You might not know what they will do next.

You can worry that if you say anything to them about their substance misuse it might make things worse. They may start drinking more or taking more drugs. They might get angry at you; they might shout or swear.

It is understandable to find this scary. Things get ignored and things just get worse. There could be stuff happening in your home that is not healthy and not ok. You don't feel like saying anything, because you are scared.

This blog post is designed to give young people the chance to explore their feelings, and offers practical steps to help them cope with addiction in the family.

You are not alone

When you have an addiction in your family, it can feel like you are fighting a battle all on your own.

It can feel like you are the only one going through this experience. But you are not alone. Addiction affects families of every kind, not just yours.

There are young people going through similar experiences to you right across the country. Some will go to private schools, some will go to state schools, some are in families with lots of money and others are in families with not much money at all.

There might even be people in your school who are going through what you are going through.

I know how difficult it is to talk about it. I know you can feel trapped and isolated. What I really want to say again, as I think it is so important – you are not alone.

There are people and organisations who understand what you are going through.

Why do some people become addicted?

There are many different ideas about why people misuse substances and become addicted. Some people think it's a disease or an illness, others think it is behaviour that has been learnt.

It doesn't matter what the addiction is; whether it's substance misuse, gambling or something else. The effects on the family and individual are always the same.

Using alcohol and drugs might not make sense when you look at what happens to the family and the pain it causes everyone.

The truth is people don't live their life thinking 'I am going to use alcohol and drugs until I hurt all the people around me, and I lose everything.'

The adult in your life might have promised to change and not to drink alcohol or take drugs ever again only to break their promises.

When people become addicted, they tend to break promises and not to tell the truth. You can feel let down and lied to. You might not believe anything they say. All of this is unfortunately what can happen when addiction is present in a family.

You can try to make sense of it but that can be impossible and can leave you feeling frustrated confused and tired. You might be thinking that if you 'work out' why someone uses then you may be able to fix the problem and make things better.

I can clearly tell you and this is 100% guaranteed, it's not your fault. Even though the person who has a substance misuse problem may have told you it was while they were drunk or using drugs.

Addiction is often a very complicated issue and is not something which you alone can fix. Often people need help and support from professionals who know how to treat addiction, in order to get better. The good news is that it is possible to get better and help and support is available when the time is right

Whilst you are dealing with a very difficult situation it is important to remember that:

♦ You are not alone, and addiction is unfortunately affecting families all around the world

♦ Remember it's not the person with the addiction you dislike, it's the way they are behaving

♦ It is not your fault and you alone cannot fix it

♦ It is important to keep yourself safe and well

♦ It is normal to experience lots of different feelings when you are going through such a difficult time

It is ok to have lots of different feelings

When we are affected by someone else's alcohol or drug use or other type of addictive behaviour, we can feel all sorts of things.

It may feel like people are judging your family because of the alcohol or drug use. Feeling judged can lead to isolation, spending time on your own and not doing the things you would like to do.

For example, not inviting friends around to your home because you are worried your mum or dad are going to be drunk and this might be embarrassing.

You might avoid people just in case they ask difficult questions that might break your family up or make the problem worse.

You may feel split. You love the person who uses alcohol or drugs but also dislike them at the same time as well.

This could lead you to feeling guilty or ashamed. Feeling angry, responsible or frightened are all completely natural and normal responses to what you are going through.

It is essential that you understand that it is ok to feel. All feelings are normal, natural and ok. It's what you do with feelings that counts.

What you might be experiencing….

In my experience night times can be hard when all sorts of feelings are around. When you are trying to go to sleep it can be more difficult to distract yourself and you start to really think about things.

In other parts of your home you may be able to hear people drinking, shouting, arguing or slamming doors.

You might find it difficult to get up in the morning if you have had a bad night's sleep. This might mean you are late for school. You might find you are struggling with your schoolwork or you might be experiencing bullying.

You could be expected to look after you brother or sister all the time. You might feel hungry sometimes because there isn't any food in the house.

What is really important is that whatever you are experiencing you find some ways to keep yourself safe and well.

What can you do to keep yourself safe?

There are some things you can do every day to help keep yourself safe and manage what you are feeling, which can often feel very scary and overwhelming.

When you are full of feelings and need to let them out somehow you could scream into a pillow in a safe part of your home. You could try to listen to some music or an audio book. You could write down your thoughts and feelings in a diary to get them out of your head and help you to make sense of what is going on. Sometimes drawing pictures can help when we don't know what words to use.

Exercise can really help us to feel better. If you are old enough and able to, you can go for a walk or a run. If it is possible, you could meet a friend in the park for a game of football or just a chat in the fresh air. If you have a garden, you can play some games outside.

It is important you find some healthy things to do which work for you.

Remember to take each day at a time. Tomorrow will be a new day, and things can change, and they can always get better.

Talk to someone you trust

Whatever you are feeling, holding your emotions in can make you feel even worse. It's really important to talk to someone about what you are going through.

You can't cure addiction and you can't control it, but you can take care of yourself by talking about how you are feeling and what is going on for you and making healthy choices.

It's important to find someone you can trust to talk to. This could be a friend a neighbour, another member of your family, a teacher at school or a counsellor.

You have a right to be safe. If you feel really scared and unsafe and are in danger or someone you know is in danger tell someone you trust or call the police.

Currently the country is going through a lockdown. This is probably making things even harder for you. Trapped at home and unable to get a release or relief.

Some of you will be really worried about the adults in in your life who have an addiction as their behaviour may be even more unreasonable and unpredictable.

Try and think about the people and numbers you can call for help and keep those close by. Focus on something you enjoy doing. Drawing, listening to music, writing, reading or exercise.

You might even need to find a safe space in your home just to keep out of the way. If in danger make the call you need to make.

Remember you are not alone. Remember all feelings are ok and it's ok to feel. Talk to someone about what is going on – you are worth listening to.

Take care and stay safe.

This article is a combination of 3 blogs by Matt Serlin, previously published on the learning platform for Action on Addiction's Centre for Addiction Treatment Studies (CATS)

Matt Serlin has a BA (Hons) in Integrative Counselling and Psychotherapy from the University of Southampton, and a Certificate in Clinical Supervision from The Centre for Supervision and Team Development, London.

With over 25 years' experience of working in the substance misuse field in both community and institutional settings, Matt has a special interest in family interventions, and working with children affected by parental substance misuse. A trained M-PACT practitioner, Matt teaches our students about working with families and significant others, and trains M-PACT practitioners across the UK and internationally. He is also a facilitator for Action on Addiction's residential family programme.

www.actiononaddiction.org.uk

I'm an addiction researcher and therapist. Here's why promoting sober 'dry months' bothers me

An article from The Conversation.

THE CONVERSATION

By Kara Fletcher, Assistant Professor, Faculty of Social Work, University of Regina

Campaigns that challenge people to abstain from alcohol for one month – often in support of a good cause – have emerged across the globe over the past decade. Dry January officially launched in 2013 with a public health campaign by British charity Alcohol Change.

Other 'month of abstinence' campaigns have included Dry July, Sober September, Sober October and 'Dry February' – a few examples of campaigns from Australia, New Zealand, the United States, Canada and beyond. Dry campaigns have gained traction with people increasingly taking a time out from drinking alcohol for one month.

Early research suggests alcohol use has increased during the COVID-19 pandemic, particularly among individuals who have mental health challenges. The pandemic may be contributing to the greater interest in dry month campaigns. Market research surveys have found an estimated one in five people participated in Dry January in 2022.

On the surface, 'dry' months are great – individuals set a personal goal to abstain from drinking, are publicly encouraged to achieve it and raise funds for a charity. It can be seen as supportive and positive, and many individuals tout the health benefits they experience as a result.

Substance use is complex

As a substance use researcher and therapist, I certainly do not dispute the potential benefits of avoiding alcohol for a month to meet personal health goals. I also appreciate the peer support received by individuals doing these challenges.

So, why was I so bothered as I listened to someone sharing the life-changing benefits of her four-week sobriety stint on the radio? Why am I irked when people express relief when their four weeks of Dry February are over, and they can get back to 'wine time?'

I'm troubled because while dry drinking campaigns benefit many, they do not help the individuals that I have worked with over the years. These attitudes and campaigns do not contribute to a more nuanced discussion about substance use. Instead, they perpetuate the idea that quitting drinking for a month is a choice, and an easy and positive one at that.

Dry February and other associated campaigns are not intended for individuals struggling with the systemic inequalities, such as poverty, illness and racism, that lead to substance use issues. You will also note that these campaigns are only about alcohol – a socially acceptable substance.

How would these campaigns be perceived if they were focused on other drugs? Dry campaigns support a harm reduction strategy – not drinking for a month for health benefits with no expectation of ongoing abstinence. However, they continue to separate alcohol as more socially acceptable than other drugs. This negatively affects people who use drugs.

These attitudes marginalise other substances and only normalise alcohol use, which contributes to the ongoing War on Drugs and deadly drug supply. Further, these campaigns praise people for not drinking, which plays into the harmful idea that drinking (and using other drugs) is bad or subversive and should be controlled.

Stigma and inequality

Arguably, these campaigns are directed at predominantly white, educated, middle class individuals who have the luxury of taking a time out from drinking, and the privilege of doing so without the risk of social stigma.

In one 2020 study comparing individuals who participated in a Dry January with the general population, those who participated in Dry January, were more likely to be younger, women, had a higher income, had completed university education and had 'significantly better self-rated physical health.'

Celebrating predominantly middle/upper-class, educated women for publicly choosing to quit drinking for one month is potentially harmful. It perpetuates an all or nothing moralistic attitude towards substance use. It reinforces the myth that quitting substance use is a choice that anyone can (and should) make.

Dry month campaigns are not directed at my clients who attend therapy for substance use issues. They do not see themselves as welcome participants in these campaigns. Their substance use or sobriety isn't trendy, or worthy of a hashtag. It's messy, it's personal and it is often much more complicated than deciding to 'just quit.' For them, drinking can be a needed self-medication tool, an endless obstacle, or an enjoyable friend.

Policy and privilege

I continue to appreciate many aspects of dry month campaigns, including raising money for charity and bringing discussions of substance use into the limelight. At the same time, these months are worthy of more critical reflection.

Substance use is complex. People often struggle with their use for reasons directly related to social inequalities, trauma, unsafe supply and poverty. Treating a four-week vacation from alcohol as a moral victory reinforces stigmatizing and negative stereotypes about people who use alcohol and other drugs. Alcohol and other drugs are not inherently bad; the policies we have made around them are what cause harm.

In the midst of Dry February, my hope for dry campaigns would be that they offer not solely a chance to examine and limit one's own drinking, but an opportunity to broaden the discussion around how privilege and policy impact one's relationship with alcohol and other drugs.

13 February 2022

Recognising addiction in yourself and others

By Emma Pawsey

We all know what an addict looks like right? It's a down-and-out person, someone without a career or home, or a washed-up rock star. Wrong. Addicts can be anyone and many demonstrate no outward signs of their addiction. The majority are employed and regularly successful, have active social lives and are fun to be around. They hide their addictions from even those closest to them. These are known as high functioning addicts.

Functioning addicts are becoming more commonplace in modern society. In particular, alcoholism is not what it used to be. Alcoholics vary greatly from moderate drinkers to those at-risk of long-term damage. Not every alcoholic or substance abuser has the train-wreck image that we imagine or is portrayed in the media. Signs of a functional addict are far more subtle and the advancement of the condition can be slower. High functioning addicts set themselves limits but inevitably go over them and are unable to quit this behaviour.

Functioning addicts in the workplace

The main trait of a functioning addict is that they maintain a successful career, therefore it comes as no surprise that many are employed in high-stress jobs, which cultivates addiction and often allows access to substances that are abused.

These careers can include:

♦ Healthcare Professionals – Doctors and nurses work under a severe amount of pressure and this intensity can make drug use an attractive option. In addition, the easy access to powerful medications makes drug use very easy.

♦ Law Enforcement – Those in law enforcement suffer drug and alcohol addiction at a rate of two to three times the national average. Similar to healthcare professionals, the availability of substances and high stress nature of the job makes substance abuse an appealing coping mechanism.

♦ Lawyers – Studies have shown that lawyers suffer alcohol abuse at a rate of twice the national average. Less conclusive were statistics regarding drug abuse, but it is considered that there are similar levels of problems within this community. The long hours that lawyers work is generally to blame; many drink excessively to cope with the stress, then take stimulants in order to maintain focus.

Am I living with an addict? How to recognise a high functioning addict

High functioning addicts are very adept at hiding their problem, usually because they fear damaging their career or reputation. There are, however, some subtle signs that may develop:

♦ Excuses and Denial – Almost all addicts deny they have a problem. The difference with high functioning addicts is that their denial can often sound acceptable. They will justify that drugs and alcohol is a reward for their hard work and success.

♦ Taking more substances than intended – We've all said 'I'll just have the one drink', only to continue drinking. However, addicts are unable to control this impulse and regularly overindulge.

♦ Their friends or family also have addiction issues – Look at the people that a suspected addict spends their time with. If they also regularly binge drink or consume substances, then it is likely there is a problem.

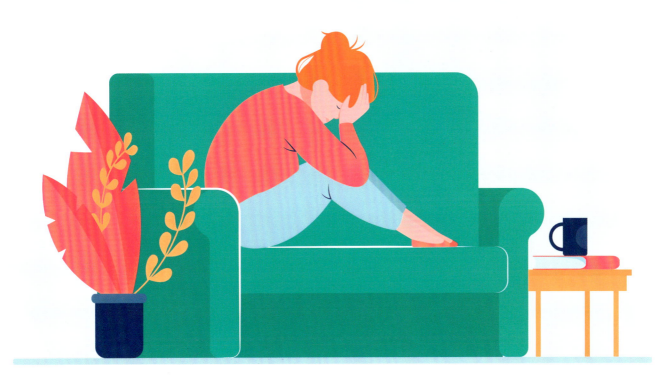

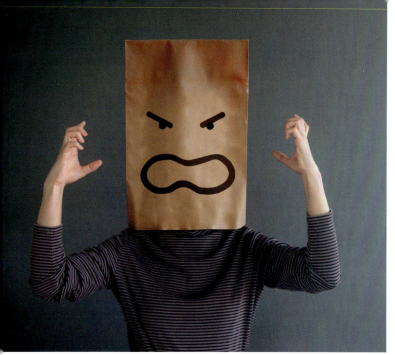

- Deteriorating appearance – A functioning addict may display symptoms such as regular headaches or lack of energy but blame these on 'not being a morning person' or similar excuses. As addiction develops further, the addict's health begins to suffer and they may not put as much energy into their appearance as usual. Look for dishevelled clothes or hair, or in the case of women, overuse of makeup to cover their deteriorating appearance.

- Losing interest in activities, becoming isolated – This usually presents in the later stages of addiction. The addict will start to withdraw from usual activities, often at short notice, which is a sign that the addiction is taking their energy and spare time and becoming a priority.

- Financial issues – Addiction is not cheap and many addicts will develop financial troubles. Because high functioning addicts are usually successful in their careers, having financial problems and asking for assistance is a particular warning sign.

- Neglecting Responsibilities – High functioning addicts are usually so successful that when they begin to neglect responsibilities this is a warning of underlying issues and a possibility that addiction is taking control of their life.

How to approach a high functioning addict

It can be very difficult to encourage a high functioning addict to get help. Many can function for years without a 'rock bottom' or life-threatening moment that causes them to face the issue. Because of the high level of denial, when the problem is eventually admitted it can be difficult to treat.

The best way to approach the subject is to start small and work your way up. Sometimes just a general conversation can be enough to 'wake up' an addict and encourage them to seek treatment.

Pick an appropriate time for a conversation, ideally when the individual is remorseful for their behaviour, not when they are under the influence or recovering immediately afterwards. It can also be beneficial to bring together a small group of loved ones to form an intervention.

Talk to your loved one about their changes in behaviour and

how this makes you feel. Point out the things that they do when under the influence and how this can cause health problems further down the line. Be prepared to be tough and remind them that although their addiction may not currently be causing problems, eventually it will, and you will not support that.

Am I an addict?

It can be harder to recognise an addiction problem within yourself than in others. Addiction is a chronic brain disease which causes permanent changes in the brain, causing you to struggle to control your impulses. Remember that addiction can happen to anyone and there is no shame in seeking help.

If you're not sure whether you may have any addiction problem, consider asking yourself these questions:

- Has your drug or alcohol use affected the relationships in your life?

- Have you ever used drugs or alcohol to 'fit in' with a certain peer or social group?

- Have you ever lied to a loved one about your substance use?

- Do you hide your substance use from others?

- Do you schedule your time around drinking or taking drugs?

- Have you tried to stop your substance use, but been unable to?

- Do you drink or use drugs first thing in the morning?

- Do you use substances to cope with stress, anger or sadness?

- Is your performance at work suffering as a result of your substance use?

- Have you been suspended or fired from your job because of your substance use?

- Have you ever partaken in risky behaviour connected with your substance use i.e. driven drunk, stolen substances or money?

- Are you concerned about your drinking or drug use?

Answering yes to some or all of the questions above may indicate that you have a substance abuse problem. Many high-functioning addicts are concerned about the effect on their career or reputation should they seek treatment. However it is important to consider the long-term benefits and how different your life can be without substance abuse.

Next steps – getting help

'I am an addict and I need help'. Once the addiction is acknowledged, it is important to seek help as soon as possible. The best place to start is with your doctor, or to contact an unbiased organisation such as The Recovery Trust who can advise the treatment options available and refer you to relevant specialists.

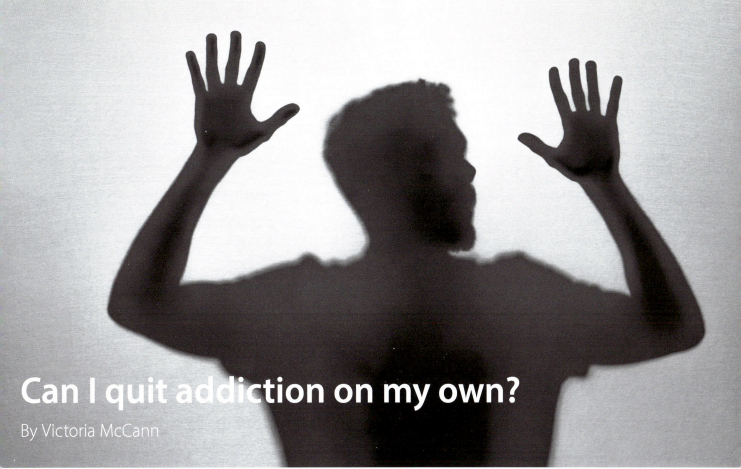

Can I quit addiction on my own?

By Victoria McCann

So you admitted you have a problem. Maybe you've proclaimed yourself as an alcoholic or drug addict, or maybe you simply think that you have developed a bad habit of drinking a few too many on the weekend. Now what? Many people, even those with a serious addiction, don't instantly jump to the conclusion of 'I need to check into a rehab tomorrow' when they realise what's going on. In fact, most people try to quit addiction on their own, in the beginning.

Even when you ask your GP or contact a community addiction centre for advice, they will give you various self-help resources to try first. Before you can get a referral to a residential rehab, you will be recommended here first. However, one needs to realise that there is a difference between having a bad habit and having an addiction. While quitting using self-help resources can be useful for some, it is not possible for everyone. In fact, promising that you can quit by yourself may be just another part of the denial process. If you think that you may be lying to yourself, or to those concerned for you, about being able to quit your addiction on your own read on for more information.

Substance abuse vs. addiction

When asking if it's possible to quit an addiction on your own, it is important first to understand what addiction is. You may have heard the terms 'substance abuse' or 'dependency' used interchangeably with the word 'addiction', but this isn't completely correct. They are all related, but they are not the same thing. If you have an addiction, this can have consequences for how hard it will be to quit on your own, and what treatment you need.

Substance abuse is using alcohol or drugs in an unintended or excessive way. Perhaps someone was prescribed painkillers after their knee surgery, and continues taking them longer than necessary. Or some people turn to alcohol in times of stress, such as bereavement. Just because someone misuses a substance doesn't mean they have an addiction. For this, they also need to be dependent on the substance. The person's mind or body feels like they 'need' their substance to go about their day.

Addiction refers to a chronic mental illness characterised by the inability to control one's habits due to cravings or withdrawal symptoms. This is a complex condition that, according to the DSM-V, needs to fulfil certain criteria of behaviour that combine substance abuse and dependency.

Someone who appears to like to drink a lot, or uses drugs recreationally, isn't necessarily addicted to the substance. Therefore for them, it may be easy to quit, because they haven't developed a physical or psychological dependency on their behaviour. It is important to recognise the difference, and establish whether you have an addiction. If you do, it will likely be more difficult to quit on your own.

Factors that affect recovery

Regardless of whether a person has an addiction or not, there are also a number of factors that can affect how easy or hard it will be for them to quit and recover. These can include:

Substance type:

Certain substances can be easier to quit than others. Some drugs, such as benzodiazepines, heroin, or even alcohol, can have prolonged and severe withdrawal symptoms that can make quitting tough. In some cases, a medically assisted detox programme is necessary.

Length of use:

The longer you use a substance, the tougher it will be to quit. This is because you will usually develop a tolerance to the substance. Your body or mind may become increasingly dependent on it and exhibit withdrawal symptoms when you quit.

Underlying problems:

A large part of recovery is understanding why you started using in the first place. Quite often, there is an underlying psychological issue, such as depression, anxiety, PTSD or a personality disorder accompanying the addiction. Without addressing it, recovery will likely be very challenging.

Genetics and other factors:

It is well-known that some groups can be more prone to addiction or have a harder time recovering. This includes women, the elderly, young adults, and veterans. Some people are also genetically predisposed to developing an addiction.

Approaches to recovery

When trying to address substance misuse, there are several different approaches one can take. Certain methods may be more effective for some than others. In addition, quite often, people will go about their recovery in stages: first, they try natural recovery or self-help methods, then they will try outpatient treatment, and finally, they will attend a residential rehab.

Natural recovery

No treatment, not even AA meetings, you just decide to quit one day, and begin a new healthy lifestyle.

Self-help

This is when a person tries to quit on their own. They may enlist their family or friends to support them or attend mutual-support groups, such as Alcoholics Anonymous or Narcotics Anonymous, but do not receive formal treatment such as therapy.

Outpatient treatment

There are many types of outpatient treatment, and they are all less intense than a residential rehabilitation programme. This can involve counselling or a day-treatment programme,

but ultimately, the person goes back to home or work, and retains their day-to-day lifestyle. This can be considered a self-help recovery approach, but with added therapy.

Residential rehab

This is the most intense treatment option, usually consisting of a four-to-six week residential programme where one lives at the treatment centre, and attends a complete treatment schedule throughout the day. When people cannot quit on their own, a residential rehab may be the best solution.

Can self-guided recovery be successful?

According to a study by the National Epidemiologic Survey on Alcohol and Related Conditions (NESARC), self-guided recovery is possible.

This can be explained by the concept of 'intrinsic motivation', when a person is not influenced by a positive or negative reinforcement factor to change their behaviour. In psychology, intrinsic motivation is considered more powerful than punishment. However, it can be extremely difficult for people with an addiction to harness this. The very nature of addiction as a brain disease means that the pleasure-reward pathway has been disrupted. There are also other factors of addiction, such as withdrawal and cravings, that be tricky to overcome.

Lastly, there are a number of situations where quitting an addiction on one's own is not recommended.

Dangers of quitting on one's own

In some cases, addressing addiction via self-help resources is not advised. Recovery involves many aspects, including detox, therapy and aftercare. In certain situations, going about it solo can lead to failure or other dangerous consequences.

With certain drugs or even prolonged alcohol use, detoxing at home is considered dangerous. Someone who has been drinking heavily for a long period of time can't easily quit 'cold turkey' and this is not recommended; in some cases it can be life-threatening. With drugs such as

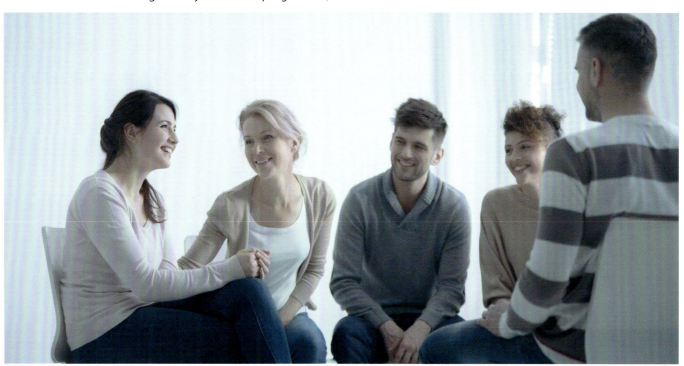

opiates or benzodiazepines, withdrawal is often lengthy and unpleasant. In these cases, they may require medical supervision or a substitute prescription.

One of the things to watch out for is developing a cross-addiction in the process of recovering from the first addiction. That means a person will trade one addiction for another. For example, somebody who tries to quit cocaine may turn to alcohol instead.

Those with a dual-diagnosis will likely find it harder to quit on their own. In professional treatment programmes, psychological problems should be treated along with the addiction. If you're going about it solo, you may not be able to address both issues at the same time.

Although relapse is quite common regardless of the treatment approach, trying to quit on one's own can result in higher failure rates. The person may use justification, such as, 'I'll have just one more drink' or 'I can minimise my use' and end up falling off the bandwagon instead.

Getting professional treatment

If you're reading this article, you may be looking for self-help addiction treatment because you want to avoid professional treatment. However, you have to ask yourself why you're doing this.

Shame and stigma often come to mind when people think about drug or alcohol addiction. You may not want to publicise that you are going into an addiction treatment programme because it'll make you look bad. You have to realise that the potential damage caused by not getting sober will likely outweigh the short period of embarrassment.

In addition, you may not want to go to inpatient facilities because of a fear you will lose your job or forgo time spent with family. Inpatient treatment may force you to take some time off to get better, but because the programmes are more intense, you will ultimately spend less time in treatment than in an outpatient or day-treatment programme.

Many people also avoid residential treatment facilities or even professional treatment programmes because of cost, thinking that these options are expensive. This is not necessarily true. There are a number of community programmes offering counselling and therapy that are free to access. Even residential rehabs don't have to cost much, or they can be covered by either the NHS or private insurance.

Self-help guide on how to quit addiction

It is possible to quit substance use or an addiction on your own, but it is not always a plausible choice for everyone. While you're in a self-guided recovery, it is wise to look into alternative options, and maybe contact a rehab centre or two about their treatment programmes. That way, when you're ready for serious treatment, you will know what to do and where to go.

In the meantime, if you are determined to try to quit on your own, try following these recommendations:

Find friends and support

There is nothing more important than having support during recovery. You will need someone (or somewhere) to go to when you have a craving, and you'll need someone you can

depend on to steer you away from temptation. Fellowship meetings and sponsors are very helpful in this aspect.

Strive for a goal

Have a large goal to strive for. For example, once you get sober, you can finish your degree and one day get your dream job! Or maybe, once you stop using, you can spend more time with your family.

Find your 'higher power'

It's helpful to have a role model or something that gives you powerful inspiration. Someone you want to impress or don't want to let down. For example, if you have children, you can always remind yourself that they'll be disappointed if you continue to use.

Build a self-care routine

Most people who quit on their own first started eating healthier and exercising. Taking care of yourself is a great motivating factor because it feels almost like immediate gratification. With an organised routine, you will start to feel better quickly, and distract yourself from cravings or withdrawal. Plus, exercise acts as a natural antidepressant.

Replacing bad habits with good ones is always a positive step.

Learn and educate yourself

Learning more about excessive drinking or the substance(s) that you're using can motivate you to quit because you'll be aware of the potential risks involved. Also, reading or listening to other people's stories about recovery can not only get you in the right mind-set but also show you that you're not alone in your journey to recovery.

Create your backup plan

Plan how long you will allow yourself to try to quit on your own, and decide what you will do if it doesn't work out. Perhaps you'll decide that if you relapse more than three times, you will immediately seek professional help. Or if your cravings are unbearable after one month, you will join an outpatient programme. Make a promise to yourself, and ideally to someone else, and stick to it.

If you do think that you need help to quit your addiction, and can't do it on your own, give us a call and we can talk about your options. We have 30 years of experience helping people overcome addiction and get into successful recovery. With our team of medical experts and professional therapists, we can help make your recovery a reality.

1 February 2019

Key Facts

- 1 in 3 people are addicted to something. (page 1)

- If your parents had an addiction there is a one in two chance you will. (page 3)

- Men are over seven times more likely than women to be addicted to gambling. (page 3)

- Treating drug and alcohol misuse costs the NHS as much as £4 billion a year. (page 4)

- 44% of Britons believe people have a large amount of control over their addictions. (page 4)

- 21% think people have little to no control over their behaviour. (page 4)

- It's estimated that two million people in the UK are currently fighting an addiction. (page 5)

- Children of addicts are 45% to 79% more likely to abuse drugs or alcohol compared to the general population. (page 5)

- The World Health Organization (WHO) controversially classified 'gaming disorder' as a disease in 2018. (page 9)

- UK teenagers are on their phones for about 18 hours a week. (page 9)

- Cocaine increases dopamine by 350 per cent; methamphetamine by 1,200 per cent. (page 10)

- 3 per cent of gamers develop problem behaviours. (page 10)

- Those aged 25-34 account for the biggest increase in online gambling of any age group. (page 10)

- More screen time during the pandemic has led to a threefold increase in myopia in children in China. (page 14)

- Gaming for more than an hour a day increased the risk of bad sleep quality by 30 percent. (page 14)

- Schoolchildren now spend an average of six hours a day in front of screens. (page 14)

- There are approximately 2.2 billion gamers across the world and the global video games industry is worth about £110 billion. (page 16)

- A group of Canadian parents have issued a lawsuit against makers of Fortnite for allegedly making the game as addictive as cocaine and 'ruining children's lives'. (page 16)

- According to WHO, about 1-3 per cent of the gaming population of people struggle with the symptoms of gaming disorder. (page 17)

- The average age of a gamer is 33 years old. (page 17)

- Around one in six people (15-20%) report addictive patterns of eating or addictive behaviours around food. (page 18)

- Children and adolescents tend to have fewer addictive eating behaviours, or symptoms, than adults. (page 19)

- Australians consume, on average, 60 grams (14 teaspoons) of table sugar (sucrose) a day. (page 20)

- Adults should have no more than 30g of sugar daily. (page 21)

- In the UK, we drink nearly 100 million cups of tea per day. (page 23)

- About 80% of coffee drunk at home is instant coffee containing around 60mg of caffeine per cup. (page 23)

- A child drinking one can of cola will be taking the equivalent caffeine intake as an adult drinking four cups of coffee. (page 23)

- up to one third of UK children, mostly young teens, consume at least one energy drink a week. (page 25)

- 54 per cent of 16- to 19-year-olds drink energy drinks, compared with an average of 31 per cent of Britons overall. (page 25)

- A 500ml can of energy drink can contain 20 teaspoons of sugar and the same amount of caffeine as two cups of coffee. (page 26)

- The energy drink industry was valued at $61 billion, with a future projection of $100 billion by 2027. (page 27)

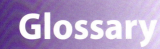

Addiction

A dependence on a substance which makes it very difficult to stop taking it. Addiction can be either physical, meaning the user's body has become dependent on the substance and will suffer negative symptoms if the substance is withdrawn, or psychological, meaning a user has no physical need to take a substance, but will experience strong cravings if it is withdrawn.

Alcohol

The type of alcohol found in drinks, ethanol, is an organic compound. The ethanol in alcoholic beverages such as wine and beer is produced through the fermentation of plants containing carbohydrates. Ethanol can cause intoxication if drunk excessively.

Caffeine

Caffeine is a natural stimulant found in drinks like tea, coffee and cola.

Cognitive behavioural therapy (CBT)

A psychological treatment which assumes that behavioural and emotional reactions are learned over a long period. A cognitive therapist will seek to identify the source of emotional problems and develop techniques to overcome them.

Detox/detoxification

To abstain from, or rid the body of unhealthy or toxic substances.

Digital detox

A period of time where a social networking user spends away from using social media. This is often to break the habit, or addiction, that some experience from using social media. Some people will also try to avoid all forms of digital communication, such as email or instant messaging in this time too.

Dopamine

Dopamine is a type of neurotransmitter and hormone. As part of the brain's reward system, it can help us feel pleasure. Often referred to as a 'happy hormone'.

Drug

A chemical that alters the way the mind and body works. Legal drugs include alcohol, tobacco, caffeine and prescription medicines taken for medical reasons. Illegal drugs taken for recreation include cannabis, cocaine, ecstasy and speed. These illegal substances are divided into three classes – A, B and C – according to the danger they pose to the user and to society (with A being the most harmful and C the least).

Gambling

An activity in which one or more persons take part, where a `stake` (most often money) is placed on the result of an event whose outcome is uncertain. Examples include betting on sporting events, lotteries, bingo or card games.

Gaming

The activity of playing games on computers, consoles or other electronic devices.

Group therapy

These are meetings for people who are seeking help for a problem and are led by trained specialists who provide professional advice and support.

Medication

If a person is diagnosed with a mental illness such as clinical depression, medication may be prescribed. Some people might not want to take medication at all and prefer talking therapies, whilst others find a combination of both works best for them.

Nicotine

An addictive chemical compound found in the nightshade family of plants that makes up about 0.6-3.0% of dry weight of tobacco. It is the nicotine contained in tobacco which causes smokers to become addicted, and many will use Nicotine Replacement Therapy such as patches, gum or electronic cigarettes to help them deal with cravings while quitting.

Rehab

A course of treatment for drug or alcohol dependence, typically at a residential facility.

Risky Behaviour

Behaviour that has the potential to get out of control or become dangerous.

Screen time

A term used to refer to the amount of time someone (usually young children) spends in front of a screen. For example, a tablet, smartphone or computer.

Social media addiction

This addiction means spending an increasing amount of time on social media, taking time away from other daily tasks. Those that are addicted experience unpleasant feelings if they cannot access their social media for any period of time. It can also affect people's sleep, as they often wake during the night to check their social media accounts.

Sugar

Sugar is a carbohydrate that is a naturally occurring nutrient that makes food taste sweet. There are a number of different sugars: glucose and fructose are found in fruit and vegetables; milk sugar is known as lactose; maltose (malt sugar) is found in malted drinks and beer; and sucrose comes from sugar cane or beet and is often referred to as 'table' or 'added' sugar. It also occurs naturally in some fruit and vegetables.

Talking therapies

These involve talking and listening. Some therapists will aim to find the root cause of a sufferer's problem and help them deal with it, some will help to change behaviour and negative thoughts, while others simply offer support.

Activities

Brainstorm

♦ In small groups, discuss what you know about addiction. Consider the following;

   • What is addiction?

   • Who can suffer from addiction?

   • What types of addiction are there?

♦ In pairs, create a list of different things that someone could be addicted to.

Research

♦ Choose one of the addictions featured in this book and do some research into how many people suffer from that addiction.

♦ Research charities/organisations that help people with addictions and create a signposting poster with them on.

♦ Create a questionnaire about caffeine. Ask people questions to find out how often they consume caffeine and how they consume it (chocolate, coffee, energy drinks, etc.).

♦ Create a questionnaire to find out how many of your peers are addicted to technology and what type.

♦ In pairs, research products that contain caffeine and list from highest to lowest by the amount they contain. Do any of these surprise you?

Design

♦ Choose one of the addictions in this book and create a poster to spot the warning signs that someone may have an addiction.

♦ Choose one of the articles in this book and create an illustration highlighting the theme of the article.

♦ Create a leaflet on how to find help and support for addiction.

♦ Create a poster to warn young people of the dangers of energy drinks.

♦ Create a poster on ways to cut down on technology use.

Oral

♦ As a class, debate the proposed ban on the sales of energy drinks for young people under the age of 18.

♦ In pairs, discuss ways that people can become addicted to something.

♦ In small groups, talk about your experience of gaming addiction. Do you consider yourself to have a issue?

♦ As a class, discuss ways in which people can become addicted to technology.

Reading/Writing

♦ Imagine you are addicted to gaming. Write an email to a friend describing how playing the game makes you feel, and how you know you need to seek help.

♦ Watch a documentary on gaming addictions and write a short review.

♦ Imagine you are an agony aunt/uncle who has received a letter from a teen who is worried about their friend who is addicted to energy drinks. How will you advise them to support their friend?

♦ Choose one of the articles in this book and write a short summary and pick out three key facts from the article.

Index

Acknowledgements

The publisher is grateful for permission to reproduce the material in this book. While every care has been taken to trace and acknowledge copyright, the publisher tenders its apology for any accidental infringement or where copyright has proved untraceable. The publisher would be pleased to come to a suitable arrangement in any such case with the rightful owner.

The material reproduced in **issues** books is provided as an educational resource only. The views, opinions and information contained within reprinted material in **issues** books do not necessarily represent those of Independence Educational Publishers and its employees.

Images

Cover image courtesy of iStock. All other images courtesy of Freepik, Pixabay and Unsplash.

Additional acknowledgements

With thanks to the Independence team: Shelley Baldry, Tracy Biram, Klaudia Sommer and Jackie Staines.

Danielle Lobban

Cambridge, September 2022